The Holistic Gardener

First Aid from the Garden

Fiann Ó Nualláin

Illustrations by Sam Chelton

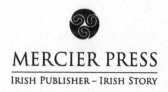

MERCIER PRESS

IRISH PUBLISHER – IRISH STORY

MERCIER PRESS

Cork

www.mercierpress.ie

First published in hardback in 2014. This edition first published in 2018.

© Text: Fiann Ó Nualláin, 2014

© Illustrations: Sam Chelton, 2014 (excluding pages 56, 91, 103, 125, 142 and 224)

ISBN: 978 1 78117 661 0

10 9 8 7 6 5 4 3 2 1

A CIP record for this title is available from the British Library

Printed and bound in the EU

CONTENTS

INTRODUCTION

Most introductions, in my experience, consist of authors waffling on about their academic status, their path to the topic and rationalising why you should be reading the book they have written. Well, let's cut to the chase here, as there is no time to waste with some topics. I have been gardening all my life, at my father's knee initially, later as a pastime through adolescence and eventually as a career after college. I have worked in the fields of amenity horticulture, landscape and design, green skills training and horticultural therapy for over twenty years, studying medical botany, global ethnobotany, herbalism, naturopathy and many holistic therapies along the way. All these extras have given me a genuine appreciation (not to mention an understanding) of the natural approach to gardening and to health – well to living, really – and that's what this book is: a celebration of gardening life and how the garden can heal you and, indeed, perhaps even save your life.

Gardeners have accidents, some very specific to the garden or to the art of gardening, and I have experienced most of them. This book gathers together my gardening and natural healing experiences to pass on to gardeners in need of first aid advice, but it is also for people who wish to use the garden and its gifts for a more natural and sustainable way of life. This book covers a lifetime of familiarity with, and knowledge about, gardens, medical botany and the trials and tribulations that occasionally befall gardeners. It is a book that incorporates practical herbalism suitable for first timers as well as practised hands – with no special skills, complicated terminology or expertise needed to master the techniques described. It is about the help that the garden can provide, although I am conscious of the need for a level of medical first aid, so I have included a section of core skills that every first aider should have and I list the traditional first aid response with each injury entry. Accidents can be traumatic or just a nuisance – discovering how to rectify the injury should not be either.

So if you have an accident in the garden (or in your home), the helpful first aid response is recorded alongside the potential for garden aid. That garden aid is further explored with carefully selected remedies that you can easily make yourself from what grows around you, plus a few items borrowed from the kitchen or bathroom cabinets. For some conditions it is good to employ techniques of functional food, and so culinary recipes extend the healing potential of both garden and larder.

A NOTE ON MEASUREMENTS AND REMEDY METHODOLOGY

The measurements of ingredients in the recipes and remedies contained in this book are not given cookbook precision. While they are highly effective, tried and tested, they are nevertheless a little more rough and ready than laboratory measurements or pharmacy doses would be – in keeping with a gardening context and the premise of the book to pick some leaves from the garden and make a quick-fix remedy – the methodology is in the spirit of grabbing a dock leaf and rubbing it on a nettle sting, or plucking a handful of thyme and pouring some boiling water over it to extract its antiseptic phytochemicals.

To work out how much dock juice diminishes the sting and how big a leaf should be to deliver that quantity, or whether a dab of antiseptic is two drops or four, only slows reaction times to treatment or complicates a natural response. A cup of camomile tea will calm or be antibacterial whether it has been steeping for 3 minutes or 30 – that said, if a herb takes a particular amount of time to disperse its health-giving properties into hot water, alcohol or an oil base, then that time will be stated in the method (steep for 10 minutes, leave for two weeks etc.).

In terms of portion size, I use 'cup' as a measure of volume, whether dry or liquid, but the metric equivalent of the American cup is 236.6ml, while what is often referred to as the 'British standard teacup' (imperial measurement) is 250ml liquid volume. We are not making soufflés or mixing dangerous substances, so for our purposes that sort of difference is not a problem. The recipes are put together by ratio method, so while I use a standard 250ml cup (not a 'World's Sexiest Gardener' mug or a bucket with a handle), the proportions of the cup you use will transfer easily enough across the board.

In culinary terms, the rule of fresh versus dried herb is that one part of dried herb is equal to three parts fresh – a good rule to follow, because even though that relates to potency of taste, it does on balance also relate to the potency of other active ingredients. Sometimes, however, drying a herb removes the volatile oils, and some phytochemicals also diminish, so fresh is always preferred. 'Fresh' will be stated in recipes where this is applicable.

Fiann Ó Nualláin

GLOSSARY

ASTRINGENT: a tightening agent, causing contraction of body tissues, checking blood flow, or restricting secretions of fluids.

COMPRESS: a pad of absorbent material or a cloth dressing moistened with an active ingredient (antiseptic, cool water, etc.) pressed onto a part of the body to relieve inflammation, agitation or to stop bleeding. A leaf or petal can also be used as a compress, such as a dock leaf to alleviate the sting of a nettle or calendula to soothe skin irritation.

DECOCTION: the liquid resulting from the extraction of the water-soluble substances of medicinal plants by boiling.

HERBAL RINSE: the herbal equivalent of a medicated wash. A cooled infusion utilised to clean a wound or alleviate a skin irritation.

INFUSION: the liquid result of steeping plant parts in hot water for 5–10 minutes.

LINIMENT: a medicated liquid applied to the skin to relieve pain, stiffness, etc.

NERVINE: a plant-based remedy that has a beneficial effect on the nervous system.

ORAL EXTRACT: any extract that can be taken orally – tea, tisane, tincture, etc.

POULTICE: a moist and often heated application for the skin consisting of substances such as kaolin, linseed or mustard, used to improve the circulation, treat inflamed areas, etc. A simple poultice employed as a drawing agent for splinters is bread dipped in hot water. A compress of steamed, crushed or otherwise prepared herbs, foliage or flowers employs both the action of a poultice (drawing/soothing) together with the application of the beneficial phytochemicals in the plants, for double effect.

SPIT POULTICE: a poultice macerated in the mouth and spat onto a wound.

TINCTURE: alcohol-based remedies for oral consumption or to be used as a rub.

TISANE: see infusion.

TOPICAL: for application to the body's surface.

INDUCTION

Yes, induction, but none of the dictates of health and safety here; hard hats are not required. This section is a guide to using the book, by looking at five core elements: what is garden aid – a brief on what is possible from the garden; what is first aid/first response – a look at the limits and practice of first-aiding; contacting emergency services – the vital numbers; a word of warning – every book needs at least one (but I also include a note on ingredients and ethical choices – not so much a warning as suggestions to give you options); and finally, and perhaps the most helpful, five steps to avoid accidents – prevention is always better than cure! (Apart from the chocolate cake cure, but more on that later.)

WHAT IS GARDEN AID?

Garden aid is a term I use to describe the use of the resources of the garden – the site of many of the accidents and injuries described in this book – to address the damage with immediate effect and often more successfully than conventional treatments, but for the most part used as a back-up treatment or 'second aid'. Think of it as a harvestable complementary therapy, as help from the garden, from its plants and the innate medicinal properties contained in flowers, seeds, leaves and sap, for injuries suffered there or elsewhere.

The plants listed in the book are not exotic or rare; they

11

are the common and popular herbs and ornamental perennials found in the average garden or garden centre. They are easy to find, easy to grow and maintain, easy to harvest and use, and are sometimes supplemented with popular herbs and spices to be found in most kitchens and local shops. And in the interest of exploiting everything the garden has to offer, I include some remedies that employ 'weeds' – I am sure you will be able to borrow some of these from a neighbour!

In this book there is a mix of scientific 'medicinal botany' and received gardeners' lore, or 'ethnobotany', about plant uses. Most people have learnt that a dock leaf cools the sting of a nettle leaf – we received that wisdom in childhood and it is part of our cultural upbringing (our learned ethnobotany) – but do we know that it is the histamine and serotonin reactions to the sharp hairs of the stinger that cause the irritation, and that dock leaf sap contains a natural antihistamine, or do we just trust that it works? It works either way. This book is not about belief, cultural norms or placebos – it is about what works. I am a holistic gardener and I do believe that gardening is prayer, but I am not of the mind to pray for rain when my beard is on fire – I will roll in the dirt and dig a plant from the soil to make a soothing balm. Using all practical skills is my kind of holistic.

So the plants selected for inclusion in garden aid are those such as the dock leaf – passed on to each generation by word of mouth while having a scientific explanation for the 'cure' effect, as well as plants from traditional herbalism, phytotherapy and pharmacognosy, studied and laboratory tested for active principles. Many over-the-counter medications for injuries listed in this book owe their origins to a plant, if they are not, indeed, outright derivatives of one. Aspirin owes a debt to the chewing of willow bark, while counter-irritant rubs for muscle aches are often derivatives of menthol and camphor extracts from garden mint, other *Mentha* species and the camphor tree. It is estimated that there are at least 120 distinct chemical substances extracted from plant sources currently employed in the manufacture of commercial drug therapies and medicinal products, and this number is growing all the time – if you'll forgive the pun.

So garden first aid is not snake oil or new age hokum, it is the most ancient, ever-renewed and certain future of healing. Better still, it is what is to hand when you need it most. You don't need to run to the pharmacist for a topical antiseptic when a natural one is growing by the knee you just grazed – for an example of this, try out the thyme antiseptic remedy on page 99.

WHAT IS FIRST AID/FIRST RESPONSE?

I list the first aid protocols for each injury under 'First response' because that is what first aid is all about – your immediate initial response. In some cases there is not much more to be done, as the job is completed with those first simple steps. But other times, or with more serious injuries, the need will arise for a 'second' opinion from a doctor, or indeed a 'second' intervention by medically trained professionals from the emergency services – paramedics, fire brigade and so on. Your first response is just the beginning of the story in that case; it is, however, if carried out diligently, the beginning that might well ensure the casualty's outcome has a happy ending.

First response is what you can do to prevent the escalation of injury to calamity level. Staying calm and focused is the best first response. There is a *universal procedure* to follow with accidents, an order of priority in an accident or emergency situation:

1. Alert the emergency services;

2. Check for danger before you proceed;

3. Do ABCs (that is, check Airway, Breathing and Circulation) on the casualty;

4. Stop any bleeding and address injuries as best you can until an ambulance arrives.

And we can add a fifth for good measure – offer reassurance/ support or, if you are the injured party, remain positive and panic free. For those who wish to explore more traditional first aid techniques, I have included a core skills section at the end of the book, covering the essential skills of taking a pulse, CPR (cardiopulmonary resuscitation), sling making, splint making and so on.

CALLING THE EMERGENCY SERVICES

Calling the emergency services may be the most important thing you do. And knowing how to do it cuts to the chase and gets vital assistance promptly to you and the casualty.

Dial 112 or 999? The well-known 999 is still active in both Ireland and Britain, as is the common European emergency number 112.

The European emergency number, 112, is the number to dial in the majority of European countries, but always check before you go on holiday to make sure that you know the number for the country you are going to.

Remember, when calling emergency services in an accident situation, 'remain calm, remain focused and remain on the line'. If using a mobile, speakerphone mode is good as it frees up your hands and you can be talked through a procedure if need be.

Always state clearly the emergency service you require and the nature of the accident. Give your name, specific location (for example, back garden, no. 16 Green Avenue) and telephone number so that the emergency services can reach you directly.

A WORD OF WARNING

Garden aid is not necessarily applicable to every situation – severe burns and serious injuries need hospitalisation – but it can be used in conjunction with best medical practice, *not instead of it*. It is not intended to take the place of traditional techniques of first response and recovery, but to support both processes where fitting; for example, a styptic (astringent) herb under a cotton pad to stop bleeding, or using immunity-building herbs in the weeks after the injury.

Misdiagnosis can be fatal in a medical situation; and in horticultural therapy or botanical medicines, misidentification can be detrimental – **knowing what you are about to harvest is what it is meant to be and is intended for the task at hand is vital**. Take time to familiarise yourself with the plants mentioned in this book – most are straightforward and generally well known, but if you supplement your garden aid from other sources then correct identification, correct application and correct dosage are vital.

So the word of warning – as promised – is 'appropriateness'!

INGREDIENTS AND ETHICAL CHOICES

To match consumer expectations and commercial consistency/viscosity within the remedies, I have elected to use items such as petroleum jelly, or emulsifying solutions such as Silcocks base or E45 cream, etc. As these are by-products of crude oil, some home crafters and ecological gardeners may have reservations about how those products might impact on oil reserves and other environmental matters. It's a complicated debate – does a by-product contribute to the damage its prime-product triggers? However, there is no health issue with these products if used in the short term for first aid, and most natural cosmetic and herbal medicine makers employ them freely. If these issues cause you concern, simply use zinc ointment, shea butter, cocoa butter or coconut oil in their place.

INGREDIENTS AND CURRENT HEALTH STATUS

Not every remedy in this book will suit everybody; for example, people with an allergy to Asteraceae plants should avoid chrysanthemum tea or oxeye daisy remedies – yet to others these may be perfect choices. The remedies in this book are based on traditional treatments and are ones I use personally, but they do not, or more to the point, *cannot* take into account the variety of individuals' underlying conditions/ current prescription medications and so on that may interact with them. So with all conditions, if you are not sure of the plant or your tolerance of it, then consultation with a qualified herbalist or naturopath is recommended. Apart from this aspect, all the usual rules apply – caution must be exercised in the case of pregnancy, high blood pressure, treatment regimes for long-term health conditions, etc.

FIVE SIMPLE TIPS TO REDUCE THE NEED FOR FIRST AID

- Avoid working in haste or under impractical time constraints. For example, do not start to mow the lawn 5 minutes before you have to collect the children from school.

- Do not attempt shortcuts – such as lifting the mower to knee-height because the strimmer is out of fuel.

- Upskill or do a little research. Many accidents are caused by a lack of skill or training to ensure that the job is done safely. Arrogance about knowing it all is as bad as knowing nothing at all.

- Be aware: ignorance of potential risks is the catalyst of calamity. Run through potential hazards before you undertake a task or project.

- Be prepared, not airlifted. A lack of planning and preparation is the downfall of all. Don't wash garden paving on nights with a frost warning and then skid the length of the newly formed patio ice-rink in the morning.

Humour aside for a moment – check out 'ergonomic tips of the trade' on pages 184–5 to help avoid garden maladies and prevent many garden accidents.

ACCIDENTS, AILMENTS AND GARDEN- RELATED CONDITIONS

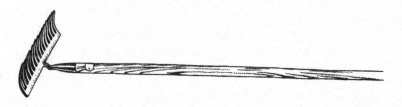

ANIMAL TO HUMAN DISEASES/ZOONOSES

A zoonotic disease is one that can be passed from animals to man. The big ones – those that hit the news or the history books – have been the plague from fleas on rats, Weil's disease from rodent urine, malaria from mosquito bites, Lyme disease from ticks, rabies from dog bites, toxoplasmosis from cat faeces and, of course, Asian bird flu and feline H5N1. Then there is ringworm and a variety of fungal diseases that seem innocuous in comparison but are nonetheless unpleasant.

Both wildlife and domestic pets can be reservoirs for infection, but even without physical contact such as hugs (passing on ringworm and other parasites), scratches (leading to cat scratch fever) or bites (possibly causing tetanus), animals can infect soil and garden plants by using your raised bed as a litter box or your shrubs as a urinal.

As a gardener, the one that concerns me the most is Weil's disease – it is a potentially life-threatening disease that is easily contracted through water barrels, ponds or even wet vegetation that has been contaminated with rat urine. Rats can also transmit salmonella, but Weil's disease can infect via not only cuts or scrapes, but also through the lining of the mouth and the tissue of your eyes – a splash can transmit it.

The time between exposure to a contaminated source and becoming sick is generally two days to four weeks, but there have been examples, where direct rat contact occurred, of the disease developing within hours. The illness manifests in two phases. The first involves fever, chills, vomiting or diarrhoea, jaundice-like appearance, headache and muscle aches. Some people only get to phase one and the illness fades out or is successfully identified and treated. A relapse or second phase is more severe – often with more pronounced jaundice, pain and symptoms that can lead to kidney or liver failure, or even meningitis. Recovery may take several months or it can be fatal.

FIRST RESPONSE

Wash the wound/contact site with plenty of water and soap to flush out bacteria/contaminants, apply antiseptic and seek medical attention as quickly as possible.

GARDEN AID

Use the phytochemicals and nutrients in the plants you grow in your garden, stock as kitchen herbs or readily source from a local health shop, to boost your immune system. Most potent are gingko leaf, astragalus root, bell peppers and other capsicums, cat's claw, echinacea, garlic, ginseng and turmeric. Barberry (bark, root and berries) is very effective against *Vibrio* bacteria and the parasitic organisms that transmit viral and bacterial infections, while goldenseal and peony can help to increase white blood cells to fight infection and viruses. The latter three are all garden centre staples, if not growing already in your garden, and all can easily be used as a tisane or tincture.

Goldenseal Tea and Tincture

Goldenseal has been used in Native American cultures for centuries, if not thousands of years, as a bitter agent, brewed or infused then ingested to stimulate the secretion and flow of bile, or applied to the skin surface as a topical solution to treat bacterial, yeast and fungal infections. It is remedial to intestinal parasites and useful as a detox herb. Goldenseal contains a good quantity of berberine, a substance also used to trigger uterine contractions and can increase blood pressure, so avoid its use in pregnancy or with conditions such as diabetes, hypertension etc.

Goldenseal tea

Roots can be harvested and dried in any season that enables correct identification, or the dried herb can be purchased from your local health store.

METHOD

Add 1 teaspoon of the dried root or store-bought herb to a cup of boiled water and allow to steep for 15 minutes. Strain off solids and drink the liquid tea. The treatment dosage is generally three times per day.

Goldenseal tincture

Tinctures are alcohol-based remedies for oral consumption or to be used as a rub. A tincture is as much a dosage as it is a preparation – usually 10–20 drops of a Mother tincture (the undiluted original potion) in a glass of spring/mineral water. The ratio for the tincture is traditionally one part herb to five parts alcohol.

METHOD

Measure out your harvested root and alcohol in this ratio and mix them together in a clear bottle or jar. Vodka or brandy works for both rubbing and oral consumption, while a remedy made with rubbing alcohol is strictly for topical application only. Leave the jar to sit on a sunny window sill for four weeks before sieving away the solids. Use the tincture fresh within two months, or decant the liquid into a dark glass container for long-term storage – tinctures are often considered to have a shelf life of ten years or longer, but I prefer to re-make if the mixture is older than eighteen months. I like to put the ingredients in a blender at the start – I feel that the blitzing releases more of the active ingredients into the alcohol base. Over the four weeks the solids separate out nicely. The traditional dosage is usually 2–4ml in a glass of water or juice, two to three times per day. Goldenseal tincture can also be dabbed onto infected areas or used in homemade ointments or salves – simply amend any salve recipe (see, for example, page 86) to include 20–40 drops of the tincture or infuse the oil base intended for the salve with plant parts for a week or longer prior to making up the salve.

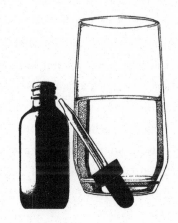

ANIMAL BITES AND SCRATCHES

ANIMAL BITES

No matter what the animal, whether it is your neighbour's pet dog or a startled fox, all animal bites carry a high risk of infection, so medical supervision is vital. If the skin is even lightly broken there is potential transmission of rabies, tetanus and a whole range of diseases and viral infections. If the flesh is torn, then professional stitching and medical intervention with wound management is essential. Do not wait for symptoms to arise. For a minor injury, see a GP the same day. For a major injury, call an ambulance or go to the accident and emergency department (A&E) of the nearest hospital.

FIRST RESPONSE ⊕

For minor wounds where the bite barely breaks the skin, wash the wound site with soap and water, apply antiseptic and visit a GP to be on the safe side – to assess the casualty's tetanus status if nothing else. For bleeding 'skin-break' bites, if the bleeding is not heavy, wash the wound with soap and water, bandage or cover it and seek professional attention as the patient may need an antibiotic and possibly a tetanus booster. Deep or serious wounds should always be cleaned and treated by trained medical personnel, so if bitten deeply, bandage the site to stem blood loss and get help from the emergency services – the patient will need an antibiotic course and a tetanus assessment.

Infection post-bite – if signs of swelling, stiffness, redness, increased pain, pus or other oozing are noticed, then see a doctor immediately.

GARDEN AID

Many of the homemade antiseptic remedies in this book (see page 99, for example) will help with bite wounds in the context of initial cleansing and later in recovery, but I seriously advise a medical examination once the wound site is cleaned up. Antiseptic plants include calendula, goldenseal (root), horseradish (root), lavender, sage, tea tree, thyme and yarrow.

KITCHEN AID

Fresh from the garden or larder, cabbage and other brassicas contain rapine, a natural antibiotic that is great in the form of a poultice. Just lightly steam a brassica leaf or quickly soften it with a touch of boiling water, and once cooled enough to place on the skin, apply to the wound site.

Echinacea Tincture

Used for internal immunity boosting and external antimicrobial action, this is one you can add to your daily beverages – a few drops in your morning orange juice, a few more drops in midday coffee. Used neat, dabs of the tincture can be applied directly to cleanse around a wound site.

Echinacea root is best, but leaves, stems and flowers are all valuable for extracting immunostimulant and antimicrobial agents. An alcohol base (500ml of vodka or brandy) is required to extract the alcohol-soluble caffeic acids, hyaluronic acid and the volatiles that are most beneficial to antibody efficacy. The fresh root has more potency, but you can obtain the dried root in most health shops and supplement this with your home-grown flower tops and some leaves.

METHODS

The slow (*menstruum*) method

Take half a cup of fresh, washed and chopped root and place it in a jar or glass container that will hold the chopped plant material and 500ml of vodka snugly. Cover with a lid. Shake the container, and label with the date. Leave to sit for five weeks at room temperature, shaking occasionally. After five weeks, strain the mixture and store the liquid in a dark bottle for long-term storage – it will keep for several years.

The quicker (*blitz*) method

Use the same ingredients blitzed in a blender, jar up and place on a sunny window sill, shaking daily, for one week. Let it stand for a second week, then strain away the solids and bottle as above.

DOSAGE AND DURATION

10–25 drops of the tincture, three times daily for five days with a short break of two days before a second round. (Rest assured this is less than a spoon of alcohol – some prescription cough bottles, antidepressants and antibiotics have more negative impact on vision and coordination than this!) Echinacea requires a break in usage to be fully effective for longer treatments. I like to time it as 'weekdays on, weekends off'. A month's treatment will make sure that phagocytosis (how the body actively eliminates invading microbes) is strengthened and accelerated, and this time frame will boost overall immune response too.

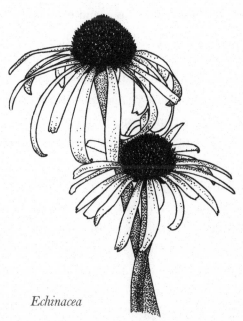

Echinacea

ANIMAL SCRATCHES

Cat scratch fever is perhaps the most publicised of the various diseases that can be transmitted via a simple scratch from your own tabby as much as from any feral tom that surprised you when you went to put out the bins. It is transference of the bacterium *Bartonella henselae* into the bloodstream via the skin break that does the damage, and the injury includes wound infection with fever, fatigue, headache, diminished appetite and swollen lymph nodes.

But it can get even more complicated, depending on your immune response. Any scratch can be an entry point for infection, but animal scratches carry a much higher risk, including rabies or tetanus – and even if you know the immunisation status of the animal in question, let's just say that animal paws are not the most sterile. If the scratch was from a wild creature then medical supervision is even more vital. As with bites, I advise you not to wait for symptoms, but apply a first response remedy and then get the scratch checked out or at least investigate your own immunisation status.

FIRST RESPONSE

For a minor wound (abrasive scrape), where the skin is barely broken, wash the wound site with soap and water, apply antiseptic, cover and protect from secondary infection. For more lacerated scratches with bleeding, if the bleeding is not heavy, wash the wound with soap and water, apply antiseptic ointment which may seal the bleed and start to tackle potential secondary infection, and bandage or cover the wound. Keep free of contamination. If bleeding is heavy, stem the flow and visit the GP or, if needed, A&E for wound assessment and possibly stitches.

Post-scratch infection – if you notice swelling, stiffness, spreading redness, increased pain, pus or other oozing, see your doctor immediately.

GARDEN AID

Many of the antiseptic remedies here will help with scratch wounds but you may, even with superficial scratches, need an antibiotic course and a tetanus assessment – so get a GP to check over the injury, on the same day if possible. Pot geraniums and pot marigolds have antiseptic attributes, as do peppermint, rosemary, sage and lavender – simply crush the leaves and rub the resulting juice over the wound, which works from the outside in, or make a simple infusion by steeping plant parts in hot water for 5–10 minutes, which works from the inside out.

Anti-infective Gels

For animal and garden scratches

METHODS

Instant gel (for same-day treatment)

Put a teaspoon of warmed petroleum jelly or zinc ointment into a shallow bowl and add 10 drops each of store-bought tea tree, clove and lavender essential oils, stirring well together. The gel can be stored for several months but is best when made fresh. Having washed the site of the scratch with soapy water, use the instant gel as an antiseptic wound ointment.

Seasoned gel

Begin with a quick tincture method – to a blender add 1 cup of mixed tops of lavender, calendula, yarrow, goldenseal and echinacea. Cover with 100ml of witch hazel extract (store-bought, or see page 188 for instructions on how to make your own) and 200ml of vodka. Blend to fine particles, then decant into a glass preserving jar (Mason or Kilner jar) and place in sunlight for two weeks. After two weeks (four is even better if you can wait) it's time to make the gel. Strain the tincture through a muslin cloth into a clean jar and discard the remaining solids. Warm the clear tincture in its new jar by placing it in a pot or basin of pre-boiled water – it needs to be warm enough to dissolve some sachets of vegetable gelatine but not too hot to hold a finger in it (which would evaporate off the useful alcohol). It may take 2–3 sachets of gelatine to reach the consistency of gel you prefer. It will store for two months in the refrigerator. Before it sets you may add double amounts of the essential oils from the instant gel recipe above to extend its potency and shelf life.

OTHER USES

While the remedies in this book are targeted at specific injuries, many are multifunctional resulting from the complexity and rich properties of their phytoactive and other ingredients. So it is worth noting that the seasoned gel makes a brilliant foot refresher after a long day of gardening, and the instant gel is excellent for chapped hands and dry elbows.

INSECT BITES AND STINGS

Most gardeners will not make it through a summer without a bite or a sting of some kind – it is an occupational hazard. But just like carpenters with splinters, one cannot fear the wood. Be vigilant about insects that bite and sting – but if you were to check under every petal and leaf before watering or weeding, the garden would soon falter.

Most insects will rush away when disturbed and are as afraid of you as you may be of their defence – and it is in defence that they sting or bite, so let them go about their business and they will leave you to yours. That said, on the other hand, some creatures (ants in particular) are hyper-defensive and relish the war more than they cherish their lives – those guys may just have to go (there are organic methods for making colonies disperse – cider vinegar for one, and borax powder if you can locate it locally, for a second).

INSECT BITE OR STING?

So, how do you know whether you have suffered a bite or a sting? Sometimes you just don't know if that sharp nip was a bite or a sting, as you only notice the inflammation later. How can you tell the difference, and how do you treat the different injuries?

A *sting* is generally an attack or defensive strike by a venomous insect, such as a bee pumping venom for 20 minutes, or a flurry of punctures by wasps or hornets, which are repeat stingers. Bees leave their barbed stinger embedded in your skin, while wasps and hornets have sabre-like stings that inject painful venom with each piercing. The stings of insects for the most part are strongly acidic or sharply alkaline, which causes the burning or 'stinging' sensation.

Bites, on the other hand, tend to be caused by non-venomous insects which, in defence or to feed on your blood, will sink their fangs or activate their mandibles to pierce your skin. Your body's natural defence to this attack is to release histamine, which triggers intense itching and causes swollen weals or hives.

There are anomalies, of course – ants both bite and sting (I told you they are aggressive!). Technically, they spray you with formic acid, which 'stings', but they often bite as well. And depending on where in the world you are, or where you bought those bananas this morning, there are biters that deposit venom too, and there are caterpillars whose hairiness causes physical (skin embedding) or allergic itch. So all is not that simple, but to make it a little easier for you, here are lists of some common stingers and biters:

Stingers
Ants
Bees
Wasps
Hornets

Biters
Ants
Fleas
Midges
Gnats
Horseflies
Ticks
Mosquitoes
Spiders

First response ✛

Search for any sting and remove it carefully. Wash the area well with soapy water and apply a proprietary or garden-sourced antiseptic.

Garden aid

To a bite or sting, apply the common weed plantain as a compress, juice dab or spit poultice (chew a bit of leaf and spit it on). A drop of mint juice is also beneficial. A mint spit poultice is therefore also an excellent choice.

Alternative aid

A tirade of expletives is said to numb pain receptors/perception. Whether or not that's true, standard toothpaste is counteractive to both sting and bite as an anti-inflammatory and to dry hives. Essential oil of lavender cools and promotes healing, as do some drops of tea tree – both great for preventing infection.

Ant bites

All ants have the capacity to bite. The common garden variety, the black ant, has no stinger in its tail end but it does have mandibles (big pinching jaws) that we may experience as a stinging sensation when an ant bites us. Black ants are never too far from aphids (which you could say they 'farm' for the sweet 'honeydew' secretions) and often among the juiciest strawberries, so a nip is not implausible, but for the most part they are not aggressive.

Their nip may be accompanied by a spectacular secondary

defence mechanism – venom, comprised mainly of formic acid and sprayed at its enemies and prey, and onto gardeners' skin. The venom has a pH ranging between 2 and 3, which makes it quite a strong acid and being sprayed is not a pleasant sensation.

An ant bite manifests as a pink, pimple-like spot of itchy irritation and often (especially with venom) as a blister-like welt or pustule. This will settle within a few hours and completely resolve naturally in a couple of days at most. Some people are allergic to ant bites and stings, however; see anaphylaxis on page 210.

FIRST RESPONSE ⊕

Rinse the bitten area under cool running water, to cool the inflamed bite and wash away any venom. Elevate the bitten limb and apply a cold cloth compress – a dampened facecloth or tea towel popped in the freezer for a few minutes works a treat. I recommend homemade calming lotion (see page 57) but over-the-counter 'anti-itch' medications will address secondary symptom relief. Try not to break any pustules, to prevent potential secondary infection. Keep the wound site clean. If there is persistent or severe swelling or itching, taking antihistamines for one to three days will resolve the problem.

Top tip

Bicarbonate of soda will neutralise formic acid. Dust some on the bitten area or make a paste with a drop of water and spread this on.

Garden aid

Gather some lavender and calendula flowers and make a strong tea, cool it and then apply as a bite-relief rinse. Make a quick salve by mixing the same flowers with a little coconut oil in a mortar and pestle, or by using the essential oil of each of the flowers in a little petroleum jelly or zinc ointment. See also the calming lotion recipe on page 57. On-the-spot first aid: the juice of succulents and the juices of plantain, chickweed and basil similarly alleviate discomfort.

Ant stings

Not all ants sting in the true sense – most do not have a physical stinger, but they do have a defence mechanism of a venom spray, discussed previously. One ant that is no stranger to the garden setting that *does* have a physical sting, however, is the red ant, often called a fire ant, not on the basis of its colour but via the burning sting it delivers with acidic venom.

Fire ants are aggressive and fearless creatures, and I say creatures because gardeners always experience them in the plural – they are never alone in an attack, so expect multiple stings. A single fire ant can deliver up to seven or eight stings in a circular pattern, injecting its toxin-rich venom with each plunge. Fire ant stings inevitably blister into white pustules accompanied by itching and irritation that can last up to a week, but most symptoms naturally resolve in a few hours to

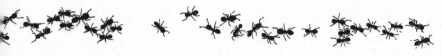

a day or two. Some people are allergic to ant bites and stings; see anaphylaxis on page 210.

FIRST RESPONSE

Stings are best treated by elevating the affected area and applying a cold pack or ice wrapped in a tea towel. But first, I recommend washing the site to flush away venom and then applying some bicarbonate of soda to neutralise any remaining formic acid, which will also help to dry out the pustules. Do not drain or break the pustules. Antihistamines and over-the-counter topical steroid creams are often recommended.

GARDEN AID

Make an infusion of echinacea flowers by steeping them in boiling water for 10 minutes. The flowers are rich in caffeic acid, which speeds the wound healing process and has been used traditionally to draw out poisons. The infusion is used as a wash, but can also be sipped to increase the body's natural immune system response. If echinacea is out of season, try chicory instead.

A compress of steamed and cooled comfrey leaves counteracts itching and heals the wound, while a cabbage leaf compress is both soothing and antiseptic. A mortar and pestle paste of chopped dock leaf, calendula flowers and bicarbonate of soda with a drop of water and a drizzle of honey also works.

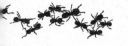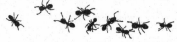

Bee stings

Bee stings are treated differently from other insect stings, as bees generally leave their sting embedded in the sting site, while other insects mostly do not. The sting site will swell up into a blister or hive and the stinger will continue to pump venom until it is removed. Once the stinger has been removed, the sting site may itch for a few hours, but overall the injury generally resolves naturally over a day or so.

First response ✚

Remove the stinger and wash the injured area with soap and water to clean and cool the site, then apply an antiseptic to prevent secondary infection. I recommend a bicarbonate of soda paste before applying antiseptic, to neutralise the acidic venom – save the dash of vinegar (most commonly and erroneously cited) for treating alkaline wasp stings.

Some people swell considerably at the site of the sting, so if stung on a finger, remove any rings as a priority. Other people can have even more severe reactions – see anaphylaxis on page 210.

Top tip

Remove the stinger and venom sac within 30 seconds of the sting to avoid receiving more venom. Use a fingernail or bank card to scrape away the stinger and sac rather than attempting to remove it with fingers or tweezers, which might squeeze or burst the sac and push more venom into the sting's puncture point. Bicarbonate of soda or toothpaste are helpful when dealing with the after-effects of the venom. Choose one of these and apply it for 10–15 minutes after washing the site of the sting. Cold therapy reduces inflammation (a chilled spoon or a chilled (used) tea bag are great options). After this treatment, antiseptic ointment or anti-itch salves can be applied.

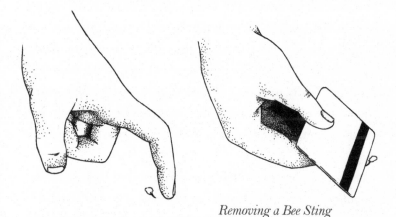

Removing a Bee Sting

GARDEN AID

A camomile tincture – flower tops and leaves slowly infused over two weeks minimum in an alcohol base – resolves any residual itching, and a mortar and pestle paste of the lawn and paving weed plantain with a pinch of salt (add a drop of water or any soothing essential oil to give a usable consistency), resolves swelling and itch. If your garden is weed-free, try grinding up basil, lemon balm or bee balm leaves with a pinch of lavender leaf plus the salt and water. See also recipes for thyme antiseptic rinse on page 99 and calming lotion on page 57.

A Bee Sting Solution

METHOD

Brew half a cup of strong camomile or lemon balm tea and instead of sugaring it add three heaped teaspoons of salt and two heaped teaspoons of bicarbonate of soda. Stir well and cool in the freezer for a minute or two – until the mixture is cool enough to use to wash the skin and begin to soothe the sting site. Return the remaining mixture to the freezer to cool sufficiently to make a chilled liquid and then dip a cotton pad or gauze strip into it to act as a cooling, antiseptic and soothing compress or use as a cold therapy rinse.

This remedy is a great itch resolver for other conditions too. It can be frozen, then thawed as required at a later date. It is particularly good for bleeding gums and oral irritations and, if the recipe quantities are increased to fill a basin, for foot blisters and toenail injuries.

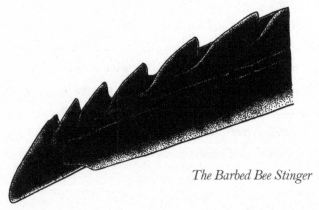

The Barbed Bee Stinger

WASP AND HORNET STINGS

Wasps, hornets and other members of the *Vespula* and *Dolichovespula* species that regularly visit our gardens have sabre-like stingers that smoothly puncture the skin, then release and puncture again repeatedly, delivering a swift inoculation of venom with each sting, and these guys can sting you several times in a matter of seconds.

The sting sites swell with the venom and histamine reaction. Similar to hives or blisters, they are sore after the sting and then become irritated and itchy. Once the sting venom is neutralised, or after it is dealt with by the body's healing mechanism, the sting swellings normally dissipate over several hours to a day or so.

Some people suffer considerable swelling on being stung by a wasp, so if stung on a finger remove any rings as a priority. Other people can have more severe reactions: see anaphylaxis on page 210.

FIRST RESPONSE ✚

Run! This is not a joke – you may have disturbed a nest and one sting will not be the limit if you have. Once safely indoors, cool the sting site(s) with tap water and then pour a little vinegar over it. There are no barbed stings to remove with wasps or their cousins, but using antihistamines will slow your body's

The Sabre-like Wasp Stinger

inflammatory response and help the venom to dissipate. Use a bag of frozen vegetables or ice in a tea towel wrap as cold therapy to numb the discomfort and reduce swelling.

GARDEN AID

A crushed basil leaf compress or squeeze of its juice is remedial to sting venom and site swelling, as are the crushed leaves of winter savory, calendula and plantain. Drink yarrow tea to counteract sensitisation by multiple stings. A mashed carrot compress is remedial.

No-waiting sting soother paste

Add 10 drops of lavender essential oil to a pea-sized amount of toothpaste and smear over the sting site to enable it to dry out. This also reduces inflammation and cools the wound.

Top tip

Wasp and hornet stings are accompanied by strongly alkaline venom. A 10-minute soak in vinegar (acetic acid) will neutralise the venom. Don't waste time with bicarbonate of soda or other alkaline substances – keep them for bee stings. You can tape on a cotton pad or strip of gauze dipped in vinegar.

Midges and nuisance insects — biting flies of the Diptera order

When it comes to midges, gnats and those near microscopic nuisances, I have to say sorry, ladies, but it is only the female of the species that bites (they feed on blood protein and males do not). However, she is no more deadly than the male, as neither of them transmits viruses or diseases, despite the pain of the bite sometimes being sharp.

Some gardeners (thick-skinned or not) don't notice the bites, but you won't fail to notice the intensely itchy reaction later on — maybe only seconds later — depending on your immune response. Those midges and gnats prefer hot and sweaty bodies to dine upon (no comment) and they secrete pheromones to let all the other flies know where the meal ticket is. So that's us gardeners (male or female) in the firing line — not just by being close to the garden but by gardening itself, whatever the ratio of perspiration and inspiration to your masterpiece.

Midges are most frequent on damp and cloudy summer days, and they do have a tendency to attack/lunch in swarms. The old saying that prevention is better than cure is apt in this case. There are many brands of insect repellent available — the more successful ones contain a chemical component called DEET (N,N-Diethyl-meta-toluamide) — but the fact that it can dissolve plastic makes me avoid it. There are many herbal repellents that contain extracts of bog myrtle or citronella and act in the same way as DEET — to disturb the olfactory sense of the insect and mask the pheromone release of the biting female midge.

First response ✚

Standard advice is 'do not scratch'. Rinse the area with fresh water, apply an antiseptic, then apply calamine lotion or similar to control the itch. Keep an eye out for infection. Bites normally resolve in a few hours to a day.

Garden aid

When the midge bites, she injects an anticoagulant into the site to enable her to feed with no time limit. Both yarrow and goldenrod are coagulating herbs – a rub of the juice from the leaves will clot those bites up and introduce agents against secondary infection. Or you could try a spit poultice of the same herbs or plantain, chickweed or basil (just chew the leaves a bit and then spit it onto the bitten area – the saliva is also medicinal to bites and secondary infection).

Horsefly bites

Horseflies are bloodsucking biters of the Tabanidae family – at least the females are during fertile periods – the peak of which coincides with warm weather and mid-summer. Their painful bites can carry disease and parasites, and in some cases fatal allergic reactions occur. In general, expect a rash and/or swelling complicated by infection, and sometimes bite reactions, even in those who are not allergic, include dizziness and/or wheezing. The big issue is that they can transmit anthrax, cholera and tularemia.

FIRST RESPONSE ⊕

Clean the site with antiseptic and take the immune response boosters detailed in this book. See a GP if you are concerned, and call the emergency services if an adverse reaction occurs.

GARDEN AID

Both mint and lemon are fragrances that deter horseflies, and yellow and royal blue sticky traps attract them (locate traps away from seating areas, open windows etc.). To eradicate them from gardens is not easy, especially if you have a pond. There are targeted chemicals available, but organically a soapy spray of one part washing-up liquid to five parts water will coat their breathing mechanism and suffocate them. Adding a clove of garlic for good measure will see a fast end to the biter.

SPIDER BITES

We tend to think of garden spiders as gardening allies and not something hazardous to our health – which they generally are, until of course one gets bitten. I am not talking here of the exotic and deadly venomous spiders that may have been accidently imported with fruit or escaped from the local pet shop, but the various species of temperate web spinners in any typical garden. The majority are not aggressive and will flee at your approach – their venom is reserved for their prey and generally is only discharged into humans when we unwittingly place our hand on one, or when they get trapped in our clothing. Most bites leave a red, inflamed puncture site that can become infected. Pain from the bite can last from an hour to several days, and the wound can last up to a week.

FIRST RESPONSE ✚

Clean the site of the bite with soap and water. Apply a cool cloth compress and if possible elevate the bitten area. Antihistamines can offer relief. Consult your GP if swelling becomes extreme or is severely painful.

On the increase are incidences of painful bites from the false black widow spider (*Steatoda spp*) – an unintentionally imported escapee with the potential to naturalise if climate change continues unabated – they are in the same family as the true black widows, but not nearly as deadly. However, severe swelling or palpitations can result from the false black widow's strong venom and a GP/hospital visit is advised in case of a more intense reaction, but in the main they are treated as a slightly more severe bite.

If bitten by a suspect species or a known harmful spider (perhaps escaped from a fruit shipment or the illegal pet trade), dial the emergency services for advice on spider identification and treatment procedure. While waiting for advice, you can cleanse the wound and slow the venom's spread with an ice pack. If the bite is located on an arm or leg, then a snug bandage (tight-ish but not a tourniquet) above the bite site is helpful, and elevation of the limb will further slow any spread of the venom.

GARDEN AID

That perennial blighter bindweed (*Convolvulus arvensis*) was once used as a strong purgative. It is currently not used in modern herbals and internal botanical medicine, but it may be helpful to the gardener suffering from a spider bite in the form of a lotion/wash made from a decoction of the leaf. A spit poultice of dock leaf is also effective, and so is a calendula compress or salve. Try any of the antiseptics explored in this book. A poultice of cooked carrots mashed with a little camomile tea is soothing and antibiotic. Arnica, witch hazel or a horse chestnut paste (blitz equal volumes of horse chestnuts to vodka or witch hazel extract) are all remedial.

Bindweed

Homemade Insect Repellents

Quick-fix midge and insect repellent

You will need 200ml of witch hazel extract from your local pharmacy (or see the 'witch's brew' recipe on page 188). Place in a saucepan with an equal ratio (⅓ cup each) of finely chopped bog myrtle, catmint and whatever garden mint you grow. Add a little fresh water if needed to cover the herbs. Put a lid on and bring to the boil, simmer for 10 minutes and allow to cool. Strain the herbs (they can be used as a bite compress) and decant the liquid into a sprayer bottle. Add 20 drops of lavender essential oil and 10 of eucalyptus or tea tree to extend storage time and boost antibacterial/antiseptic action. Store the bottle in the fridge – it keeps for several weeks. Apply as needed.

Essential bite block

Add the essential oils of citronella, eucalyptus or tea tree (all discouraging scents to insects) with rosemary, bergamot or lemongrass (also remedial and deterrent but they are more pleasant fragrances to the human sense of smell) to your sunblock or a moisturising skin cream type of carrier – the aim is approximately one part essential oil mix to fifteen parts of the carrier. I find it handy to measure in teaspoons for small batches. I prefer bergamot to lemongrass from the fragrance point of view, but you can play with the mix to produce an aroma pleasing to yourself and displeasing to the little biters. With the sunblock you get double protection.

Bog myrtle

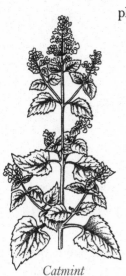

Catmint

TICK BITE

A tick is a blood-sucking parasite – a small arachnid – with the potential to transmit dermatologic infection, viral disease and bacterial infection – including Lyme disease (*Borrelia burgdorferi* or *Borrelia afzelii*). Most tick bites heal within two to three weeks if secondary infection is avoided. Be vigilant post-bite, not just for localised irritation but also for a rash, fever, muscle aches, joint inflammation, swollen lymph nodes or flu-like symptoms – if any symptoms arise, consult your GP.

FIRST RESPONSE ⊕

Remove the tick (see instructions below), wash the site with soapy water and apply antiseptic. Antibiotics are advised where the tick is suspected of being a carrier of Lyme disease.

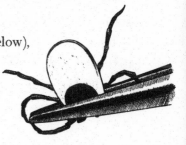

Removing a Tick

TO REMOVE THE TICK

1. Carefully use tweezers or a tick removal device to grip the tick's head as close to the skin/embedded point as possible.
2. Do not twist or jerk the tweezers but gently pull it, removing the tick intact.
3. Take care not to crush it or sever the body from the head on removal.

Despite some survivalist musings, the use of petroleum jelly, spirit alcohol or a lit match does not effectively remove a tick. If you cannot successfully remove the tick intact, consult your GP.

Top tip

If possible, save the specimen for a week – seal the tick in an airtight container and freeze for a week in case illness arises post-bite and medical staff require a sample for diagnosis.

GARDEN AID

Herbal teas of yarrow, thyme, echinacea, etc., will boost your defences and infection-fighting potential from within. They can also be used as topical washes (include lavender and mint) to fight bacteria such as staphylococcus and streptococcus associated with tick bites and in particular tick material left behind after poor removal. Camomile tea and homemade calming lotion (see page 57) will help with itching/scratching.

Specific to Lyme infection: The roots of Japanese knotweed, boiled to drink as a tea, is gaining acceptance as a long-term treatment for Lyme disease – the active ingredient is resveratrol. It can be great to supplement this with cat's claw and/or sarsaparilla products from the local health store. While the *borrelia* bacteria is routinely treated with antibiotics, it is a spirochete (corkscrew-shaped) and often bores into tissues and cartilage – so out of reach of most antibiotics. Consult a qualified herbalist about anti-spirochete herbs suitable to your constitution, which will unscrew the bacteria back into the blood stream to be dealt with by your immune system, antibacterial herbs and antibiotics.

The Sicilian Sting Thing
An offer you just can't refuse ...

I love functional food and this one hits the spot perfectly – the frozen dessert granita siciliana but with a twist – made with antihistamine herbal tea. Traditional Sicilian granita is made with sugar, water and citrus fruit juice or coffee/tea, so the flavours of our garden-grown range of herbal teas are not a million miles away.

It is a great treat for children traumatised by a summer sting and it soothes more than tears away. I am a big kid myself and one with a sweet tooth, so I keep a granita on the go in the freezer for times when I get a sting and for the odd hot Sunday afternoon too.

INGREDIENTS (PER 2 CUPS OF GRANITA)

- 1 mug strong herbal tea. I personally prefer a blend of camomile, echinacea or fennel, but you can mix and match any antihistamine herbs to suit your taste – spice it up with a little ginger, etc.
- 1 cup fruit juice – pick a flavour to supplement/complement the taste of the herbal tea(s) chosen – orange, lemon, lime, apple, or experiment with pineapple, blackcurrant, cranberry, guava, mango, papaya or even homemade cordial or elderberry lemonade – all rich in vitamin C and loaded with antihistamine action

½ cup brown sugar

1 tablespoon honey

METHOD

Make a mug of strong herbal tea with boiling water – you can use fresh ingredients in a teapot or cafetière, or use store-bought tea bags in the mug. 'Strong' is just a long soak in boiling water to extract the maximum of the active ingredients.

Make a simple syrup by combining the hot tea with the honey and sugar, stirring until the sugar dissolves. Add to the fruit juice to boost vitamin C and begin the cooling process. Stir and let the mixture sit for a few minutes.

Pour the mixture into a flat-bottomed, freezer-proof dish. I like to dust the top with a little sprinkle of sugar to start the granulation process.

Place the dish in the freezer for 30 minutes, then remove and stir/rake the mixture thoroughly with a fork. Replace in the freezer for a further 30 minutes. For the best granita, the raking process should be repeated every 30 minutes for 3–4 hours – the aim is to prevent water-ice crystals from forming and keep a consistency similar to sorbet.

You can serve the granita after 3–4 hours, or keep it frozen for a further 24 hours. After that, ice crystals will form and change the nature of the granita, but it will still be good to enjoy.

PLANT INTERACTIONS

One might be forgiven for thinking that the act of gardening – its actions – is the sole contributor to gardening injuries, but the very things we love most about gardening – our precious plants and beautiful flowers – can harbour mischief in themselves with allergenic pollen and irritant sap. Not all gardeners suffer allergic reactions, but even those without allergies are not immune to infection by a sharp thorn, or a burning splash of phototoxic sap. Some humans interact badly with certain plants, and some plants interact badly with all humans.

There are few plants that sting – nettles being a universally encountered example – but there are plenty with spines, barbs and prickles, all potentially carrying the risk of infection and disease transmission.

ANTIHISTAMINE HERBS AND FOOD

Histamine is a chemical human beings produce naturally as a defence mechanism in immune response as well as being a natural neurotransmitter. In some responses (insect stings, urticaria, allergies, etc.) it does too good a job and the defence inflammation causes as much irritation as the trigger.

Antihistamine agents serve to reduce or eliminate that side-effect. The best natural antihistamines are contained in the flavonoids that colour our fruits and vegetables, and in the phytochemicals in many herbs and edible plants. Particularly effective are plants containing quercetin, procyanidins and other bioavailable flavonoids. Below is a sample list of plants and foodstuffs rich in such antihistaminic constituents, which can easily be added to your diet when needed:

Apples	Garlic
Apple cider vinegar	Ginger
Aronia berries	Ginkgo
Basil	Green tea
Bell peppers	Kale
Broccoli	Lemon balm
Blueberries	Nettles
Cabbage	Onions
Capers	Radishes
Camomile	Raspberries
Citrus fruits	Sweet potatoes
Cranberries	Thyme
Echinacea spp	Tomatoes
Fennel	Yoghurt (probiotic/natural)

There is a wide enough range here to cover breakfast, lunch and dinner. You can supplement your daily meals with a little extra when allergies or injuries arise. And a note regarding supplements: an enzyme extracted from pineapple known as bromelain is anti-inflammatory in its own right and has the great additional benefit of facilitating a more efficient absorption of quercetin and flavonoids from the foods and herbs listed above. Also, many protein shakes contain natural antihistaminic minerals such as selenium, magnesium citrate and calcium citrate if you choose to take a smoothie/shake route to control histamine production and flare up.

NETTLE RASH/URTICARIA/HIVES

Nettle rash is characterised by sudden outbreaks of red, and generally itchy, spots or welts on the skin called hives. Medicinally, nettle rash is referred to as 'urticaria' because the hive (outbreak) resembles the sting of a nettle (*Urtica dioica*). Unlike a nettle sting, though, in about 90 per cent of cases there is no apparent or definitive cause of the rash, but it is caused by histamine production, which indicates an allergic response.

Pollen, plant sap, spores, insects, dander, some chemicals, soaps and a large range of garden-encountered substances can trigger histamine release by cells in the skin, causing blood vessels to dilate and leak fluid under the skin's surface, and this oedema is the basis of the hive/rash/urticaria.

Nettle rash usually resolves within twenty-four hours. Longer-lasting bouts are considered to be chronic urticaria and require antihistamines and a care regime.

FIRST RESPONSE ⊕

Do not scratch the itch. Instead rinse the area of rash under cool water to alleviate the hive agitation and remove potential triggering allergens (pollen grains, etc.) and then apply a calming lotion – there are many over-the-counter brands available in your local pharmacy. Most often recommended is calamine lotion, which contains zinc. Zinc is antipruritic (stops itching).

GARDEN AID

There are many garden plants and weeds that have anti-histamine principles – not least nettles – so that is easy to remember. Drinking a tea or eating the leaves will introduce the active principle into the bloodstream, and a cooled tea used to rinse the rash will speed its resolution. Likewise, yarrow, basil, camomile, echinacea, fennel, oregano and tarragon can all be eaten or applied directly to the hives. A rub of aloe vera sap, pineapple juice, burdock sap or a green tea poultice works wonders too.

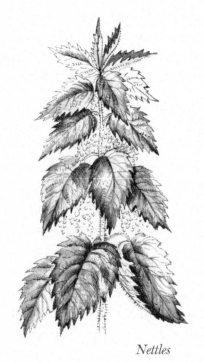

Nettles

Calming Lotion

All the ingredients here work to reduce skin inflammation and neutralise the histamine or defence reaction caused by nettle rash, nettle sting, heat rash, sunburn and other irritations.

INGREDIENTS

1 tablespoon bicarbonate of soda

1 tablespoon salt

3 tablespoons zinc ointment

10 drops lavender essential oil

1 cup strong camomile tea

METHOD

In a cup or bowl, combine the first four ingredients and stir. Then add four teaspoons of the camomile tea and mix. The water and fats of the ointment will take a good stirring to mix and become a lotion consistency. Keep adding small quantities of the tea and stirring the mixture until you have a consistency that you are happy to apply to the affected area of skin.

Keep the lotion refrigerated and use within three days of making.

NETTLE STING

Nettles, both the common 'stinging nettle' and the 'small nettle', which also stings, are common garden weeds, encountered regularly. They make their way into even the most frequently weeded garden. So many birds feed off their seeds that a dropping or two is enough to reintroduce the plant. As an organic gardener I actively cultivate nettles in a large container to harvest them for homemade nitrogen-rich liquid feed, and as a functional foodie I also harvest nettles for their array of nutritious health benefits. So a sting is a regular thing for me, sometimes even through gloves.

The thing with nettles is that their stinging hairs are in reality tiny, sharp, polished spines, so they can penetrate gloves. Those spines contain, and release on contact, histamine, methanoic acid and formic acid – three very irritating acidic chemicals. The spines may break the skin's surface and inject these agents, causing a stinging sensation and blisters. Itching and inflammation generally follow.

FIRST RESPONSE

Do not scratch the affected area. Cool with hose or tap water and use an alkaline lotion or solution to neutralise the acidic chemicals and halt the stinging action. Bicarbonate of soda works well. Follow up with a cooling lotion or salve to address the irritation and itchiness.

GARDEN AID

Acids need to be neutralised with an alkali, and the two old gardening options are a dab of urine (ammonia) or a rub with dock or sorrel leaf juice (alkaline agent). Believe it or not, the juice of the offending nettle also neutralises the sting of its hairs, if you can't find a dock leaf or a safe place to pee. Comfrey contains antihistaminic juices too, for handy topical applications.

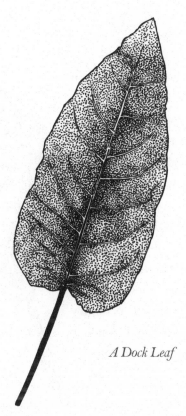

A Dock Leaf

Spit Poultice

Great for bites and stings, scrapes, cuts, bruises, blisters and burns.

A spit poultice is just what it sounds like – a poultice macerated in the mouth and spat onto the wound. It sounds disgusting but is one of the most ancient arts of healing, mixing the antiseptic potential of saliva with beneficial phytochemicals in the selected leaves – to early man and before sliced bread, it was the best thing.

METHOD

Pick the desired leaves, give them a rinse, chew on them a little and then spit them out to spread over the wound/affected area.

Suitable spit poultice leaves include bee balm, chickweed, creeping jenny, ground ivy, mint, selfheal and violet, but by far the best are plantain and yarrow. A spit poultice can be a combination of these healers. Spit poultices are remedial to sundry minor garden injuries and conditions of inflamed or irritated skin.

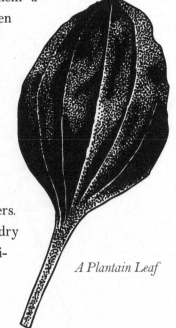

A Plantain Leaf

Phytodermatitis

Phytodermatitis is plant-triggered dermatitis. It can be acute or chronic, and is triggered by a contact allergy/sensitivity to the plant leaves, stems or roots, or sap or pollen. Plant dermatitis often manifests as a linear or streaky pattern and is nearly always asymmetrical. Some people are particularly sensitive to plants that other gardeners take for granted as being safe – such as chrysanthemums, ornamental daisies and other members of the Compositae/Asteraceae family. Some find lilies a problem, while in other cases certain trees cause flare-ups. The sap of euphorbia is a notorious culprit (yet it was once used to remove warts). In the end, it may just boil down to editing your garden of the dangers.

Plant dermatitis for the most part is considered self-limiting. It clears up without treatment once further exposure to the triggering plant is avoided, but in some severe cases it will be necessary to use topical steroids. As with all allergic reactions, some sensitivities take years to resolve, or a lifetime to manage.

Garden aid

Spit poultices and a calming lotion can be an aid, but understand your own plant sensitivities before making either of these – lest the charge becomes that of being an aider and abettor!

Kitchen aid

Vinegar and thyme washes will help with rashes and blistering.

61

Phytophotodermatitis

Phytophotodermatitis can strike any gardener. The issue lies with certain plants' sun reactive sap or other light-sensitising botanical substances. It manifests as a burning erythema (reddening of the skin) or a blistering inflammatory eruption – sometimes within moments of contact, but on other occasions it only begins some twenty-four hours after exposure. Sometimes pigment changes occur as a result of injury. It is a self-limiting condition.

Furocoumarins are one of the most active photosensitising chemical components in plants, particularly within the Umbelliferae family – including some edible plants in this group, like celery, parsnips and carrots, but not all are sensitive.

Phytophotodermatitis is often colloquially termed 'strimmer rash', where splashes of the sap of Umbelliferae weeds are sprayed about during grass-cutting or strimmer weeding – hogweeds being particular culprits.

First response ⊕

Sunlight is necessary to start the reaction, so cover the skin and go indoors, wash off the sap with soapy water and pat the affected skin dry. If a large area or the face is badly affected, consult your GP. Cold therapy is helpful for the first three days post-event.

Garden aid

As a support to system recovery, useful infusions taken internally and applied externally include willow bark or leaves, echinacea and nettle. The previously listed calming lotion (see page 57) or any of the skin benefiting treatments can be used from day two onwards for a week after the event.

ALLERGIC CONTACT DERMATITIS (ACD)

Allergic contact dermatitis may or may not be the result of plant contact, but it is helpful to explore it further here as its remedy is also useful for the two other dermatitis conditions already described. It is a reaction to a substance, material or plant with which you have come into contact; it generally manifests post-contact as an area of itchy, inflamed skin at the place where contact took place. In severe cases and where scratching is not avoided, the site can develop sores. Occasionally, a prolonged rash and auto-eczematisation can occur. In most scenarios ACD reactions disappear within days, but the reaction potential persists indefinitely.

The delayed reaction can hinder the discovery of the triggering allergen, which will need to be avoided, or removed, if possible, from the garden. The symptoms of ACD or any active dermatitis are generally treated with emollient creams. Often ACD sufferers are prescribed topical steroids and topical or oral antibiotics for any secondary infection that might have arisen. In severe cases, oral steroids or immunosuppressive medications are employed.

FIRST RESPONSE

Wash the affected area with clean water to remove any

residual allergen. I would follow with a lavender or rosemary herbal rinse to lessen irritation and swelling, and to ward off any secondary infection through their anti-microbial activity. Allow irritated skin to breathe for a day. If the irritation is not beginning to subside after that, or if this is not the first time an ACD incident has occurred, then begin longer-term treatment using a more sustained remedy in the form of a medicinal emollient or healing salve.

GARDEN AID

Use applications of aloe vera gel or strawberry pulp to cool and soothe the irritated skin as soon as it happens, or make a salve from chickweed and calendula – two excellent skin healing agents – with some evening primrose oil for extra benefit. Oral extracts of evening primrose oil and oolong tea or red peony tea are also good. A decoction of oxeye daisy is beneficial to skin, from chapped hands to eruptive complaints, including skin ulcers and cutaneous diseases.

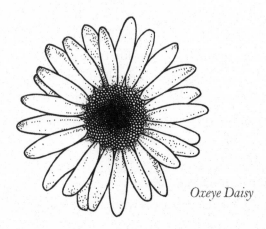

Oxeye Daisy

Geranium, Rose and Camomile Body Wash for Irritated Skin Conditions

The essential oil of pot geranium reduces inflammation of the skin and controls infection in wounds – infusions, flower essences and petal maceration (flowers, for compresses, softened with a touch of hot water or mashed to a paste in a pestle and mortar) also work well. Rose is both tonic and soothing to skin, while camomile is great for all complexion types. It is gentle on seborrhoea and helps to flush toxins from skin capillaries.

INGREDIENTS

- 1 litre distilled/spring water
- 2 cups camomile flowers
- 2 cups rose petals
- 1 cup geranium flowers and leaves
- ½ bar (approx. 50g) unscented, low allergen soap
- 2 tablespoons vegetable glycerine

METHOD

Place the floral ingredients and water in a lidded saucepan. Bring to the boil and simmer, covered, for 30 minutes. Allow to cool fully. Strain out the flowers (discard or mix them with honey to produce a face mask or skin patch). Grate the soap into the infusion and bring the liquid to the boil again, stirring until the soap is fully dissolved – hand whisking or using a hand blender is OK. Stir in the glycerine. Leave to settle overnight.

The next day, if the mixture is too thick and not the right gloopy texture, slowly add extra water or witch hazel to improve the consistency or blend again to break it up into a better density for decanting.

The mixture will store for a year but it's generally used within months, if not weeks, of making. Most natural soaps will hold a liquid soap consistency after this recipe, but some natural soaps may not be 100 per cent natural – they may have extra oils, fats, etc., in them – and so may separate into layers over time and need a good shake before each use.

The supple and subtle supplement versions

If you are not allergic to essential oils, you can supplement the natural botanical ingredients with 20–30 drops of each of their essential oil counterparts for extra potency/aroma – add at the final whisk stage.

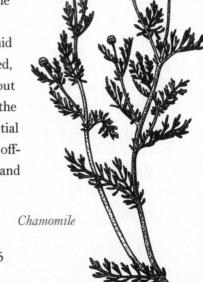

If you have a favourite liquid soap or cannot find an unscented, low allergen bar soap or are out of the flowering season of the botanicals, simply add the essential oils of the botanicals to any off-the-shelf low allergenic liquid hand soap or body wash.

Chamomile

POLLEN AND ALLERGIES

Reactions to pollen may be as severe as asthma or hay fever, or as mild as an occasional watery eye or a few unseasonal sneezes, but pollen can have an impact on a gardener's health so we need to respect the potential.

GARDENERS' PRECAUTIONS

The majority of tree pollen is released during the spring, while grass pollen is more prolific towards the end of spring and the beginning of summer. If you cannot cut the lawn regularly before it goes to seed, which is its pollen release, then remove it and plant a non-flowering camomile lawn or lay paving. Keep on top of weeds as their pollen is produced pretty much year round. Your garden plants have a range across the seasons, but summer is the danger zone. There are plenty of good choices of plants to be made – long corollas, trumpets and bell-shaped flowers hold on to most of the plant's pollen, and double blooms have no pollen at all.

Listen to/watch weather forecasts as they regularly detail the pollen count; if the count is high, give the garden a miss for the day. Consider buying wraparound sunglasses to prevent pollen getting in your eyes, and wear a wide-brimmed hat to trap particles before they reach your eyes or nostrils. Disposable face masks are a great option. At the end of the day, change out of your gardening clothes and take a shower to remove any pollen on your body, to avoid delayed reactions.

Green Tea Goo:
an allergy-free soapy body wash

To remove pollen grains after a day's gardening and give the skin some tonic and anti-allergenic properties.

INGREDIENTS

- ½ cup loose-leaf green tea, or an equivalent quantity in tea bags
- ½ bar (approx. 50g) unscented, low allergen soap
- 1 litre water
- 4 tablespoons glycerine

METHOD

Make a strong pot of the green tea and leave to cool completely. Strain away the tea solids for a clearer liquid goo or leave in for a textured fleck. Put the liquid into a saucepan and reheat to a simmer.

Grate the soap bar into the heated tea and stir to dissolve (you may need to simmer for a while, or boil up for a short time to speed up the process). Once the soap has dissolved, remove from the heat, add the glycerine and hand blend or whisk up to a froth.

Allow to rest and set overnight – the froth will settle down during this time. The next day give a second whisking before decanting into storage containers.

If the mixture is stiffer than you'd like, add some fresh green tea or hypoallergenic liquid soap while you whisk the mixture to alter the final viscosity.

Different soap bars yield different results, and some may settle in layers, but a shake before use usually solves this problem.

Quick fix

You can make a quick-fix version of the body wash by diluting a bottle of thick hypoallergenic liquid soap with a strong cup of green tea or a tincture of green tea, simply made by extracting the tea's helpful phytochemicals in alcohol (see goldenseal tincture on page 22) rather than hot water – this will take two weeks, so if time is of the essence, stick with making a quick cuppa.

Hay fever

Heaven forbid you are a gardener with hay fever or a pollen allergy – it just makes life much more difficult. But you can continue to garden – the trick is to do your gardening at low-pollen-count times of the day and year, and plant low-pollen-releasing plants (often bell-shaped) among double blooms and other sterile flowers that produce no pollen at all.

Some years pollen counts can be particularly high and even those who are not hay fever sufferers find themselves overwhelmed and experiencing symptoms including sneezing, a runny nose and watering or itchy eyes. The problem is that microscopic pollen grains are protein loaded and thus trigger inflammation in the small air-filled cavities of the sinuses as well as causing irritation to the eyes and throat.

It is often the case that childhood hay fever lessens in intensity with age and may even disappear altogether, and it may be that some adults have one or two reactions but do not go on to develop repeat hay fever.

Conventional treatment options include the use of over-the-counter or prescription antihistamines to prevent the onset of allergic reactions, and the use of prescription corticosteroids to reduce inflammation. For more persistent or severe reactions, the sufferer may consider immunotherapy – much like homeopathy, where the patient is exposed to small amounts of pollen over a long time period (months to years) to build up resistance.

GARDEN AID

Marshmallow, echinacea, eyebright, goldenrod, elderflower and cramp bark all help as infusions/tinctures to alleviate congestion, inflammation and sensitivity.

KITCHEN AID

An easy way of employing immunotherapy is to have locally produced honey in your diet; local bees will have encountered and sampled the full diversity of pollen-producing plant life in your region. Using regular small doses on your toast or sweetening your tea will build up your immunity prior to a summer flood of pollen. You may also enjoy throughout the year some herbal teas that have an antihistamine action to help prevent strong summer reactions. My personal favourites are lemon balm, camomile, fennel and echinacea.

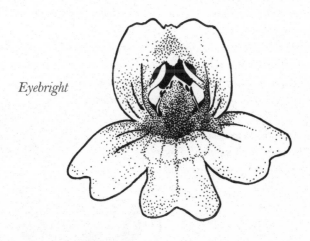

Eyebright

The Nay-Fever Breakfast – Antihistamine Tea and Toast

I am a tea and toast man in the morning, like millions of gardeners ... but we can make it functional rather than just a practical breakfast option. Simply change your tea blend. Swap the milky black tea for a green tea that reduces inflammation. Try some herbal tea: camomile has potent antihistamine properties and fennel tea is packed with quercetin – one of nature's strongest antihistamines. There is a flavour out there for you and all contain bioflavonoids that can potentially lessen histamine reactions.

When it comes to the toast, why not spread a little joy – use local honey to introduce the benefits of immunology while adding a berry jam made from your own home-grown blackcurrants, strawberries, elderberries, raspberries, etc. Get funky with the mix if you feel like it. That homemade jam has both the immunology and the antihistaminic properties of vitamin C and pectin, in one sweet dose.

If you prefer savoury tastes, why not have an allergy-easing omega-3-enriched spread with a sprinkle of thyme or oregano on top? Both Thymus vulgaris and Origanum vulgare contain a multitude of antihistaminic phytochemicals.

Last, but not least, add a piece of fruit: papaya inhibits the secretion of histamine, while oranges and other citrus fruits prevent the manufacture of histamine in the first place through their quercetin content. Add some guava, mango, peach, cantaloupe or any of your favourite fruits for their rich vitamin C content and a whole booty of helpful bioflavonoids.

Of course, berries, fruits, honey and jam all go well with muesli and cereals too. Yum!

SUDDEN POLLEN/DUST REACTION AND/OR ASTHMA ATTACK

Pollen can trigger runny eyes, wheezing and sneezing; but it can also react more intensely and cause respiratory distress akin to an asthma attack or indeed trigger an actual attack in a person with underlying asthma or a bronchial condition. Dust reactions can also catch the throat and trigger respiratory discomfort – choking, wheezing, coughing, etc. Without prior attacks one can have an asthma type of reaction in the garden through exposure to particles, hedge trimming, dusty sheds etc. Or one might have a visitor to the garden who has an asthmatic reaction.

Asthma is a long-term controllable condition of the respiratory system. An asthma attack is caused by inflammation of the airways, triggering coughing, wheezing and breathlessness ranging from irritation to debilitation. A severe onset of symptoms may require hospital treatment and can, at the extreme, be life-threatening. Common triggers of an attack include dust, dust mites, insect dander, animal fur, pollen, tobacco smoke, cold air and a reaction to a chest infection. If you are an asthmatic gardener, use a surgical mask when trimming hedges or stirring up dust. Plant low-pollen plants – those not pollinated by wind, those with double flowers (sterile), and those with bell-shaped or deep flowers where the pollen sticks to the bee and doesn't waft into the air, or plants that don't flower or spore at all – and do check forecasts for a high pollen count.

First response ✚

Assist the casualty into a comfortable, upright sitting position. If the person has asthma medication, such as an inhaler, assist him or her in using it. If the person does not have an inhaler, keep calm and reassure the casualty, advising him or her to lean forward and slowly exhale the air from the lungs. Gasping for breath can agitate the respiratory tract further, but exhaling as much as possible may filter out the triggering allergen and the natural inhalation following a slow exhalation can draw clean air in to cool the agitation. Call for someone to get an ambulance or ring for one yourself while you help to steady the casualty's breathing rhythm.

If the casualty has an inhaler, but is not relieved after using it, call the emergency services. A mild asthma attack should be relieved within 3–4 minutes after puffing on an inhaler.

Garden aid

While aromatic fragrances of common garden herbs can cool and open the respiratory system post-attack, do note that pollen and dander, etc., near plants can exacerbate symptoms. However, a herbal bath using lavender, camomile or rosemary may help regain composure and relax the body and mind.

Kitchen aid

A tea produced from an infusion of caraway seeds causes bronchodilation and can help respiratory agitation and breathing difficulties. Traditional tea and coffee both contain a chemical (theophylline) similar in action to some asthmatic medications, so after an attack a nice cuppa relaxes too.

Long before inhalers, the old folk treatment was steam inhalation, and if all else fails it can be a good alternative first aid treatment for an asthma attack. Simply boil a kettle, pour the hot water into a basin and let the casualty inhale the steam. It offers a focus, and focus calms. It also works to ease tightness of the chest and the choking sensation, which reassures further. Moist air opens the breathing pathway.

Luxury Lavender Bath Salts

A recipe using the full aromatherapeutic benefit of adaptogenic lavender and the skin healing/tonic benefits of natural salts and minerals. This remedy is not just therapeutic to skin conditions, burns/scalds, bruises and bumps, but also to aches and pains, hard days and long hours. It is also somewhat curative to the stresses caused by slug damage, ill-ripening fruits, failed propagation and that mail-order 'scarlet' rose now flowering a watery salmon pink.

Excellent to de-stress or to regain composure after any minor injury episode, taking a bath with these salts also allows you a moment to catch your breath after any incidence of respiratory distress or emotional shock.

INGREDIENTS

2 cups Epsom salts

1 cup bicarbonate of soda

½ cup sea salt

½ cup lavender flowers

21 drops essential lavender oil

A ziplock or resealable freezer bag

A sheet of baking parchment/wax paper

A Mason or Kilner jar or other similar container

METHOD

Put all the dry ingredients into the freezer bag, seal it and shake well. Add seven drops of essential oil, seal and shake. Repeat this process three times – adding all the oil at once will just gunge up the salts and soda. Spread the salts out onto the wax paper/baking parchment and allow to air dry for approximately one hour – stir the mixture after about 30 minutes. Store the bath salts in an airtight container, using as required. These salts store for months and are great to make for gifts.

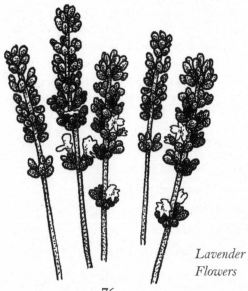

Lavender
Flowers

ROSE GARDENER'S DISEASE/ROSE THORN ILLNESS/SPOROTRICHOSIS

Sporotrichosis is an infection caused by the dimorphic fungus *Sporothrix schenckii*. The fungal spores are not exclusive to roses, also being found in hay, sphagnum moss, pine needles and wood chippings – regular ingredients of many a gardener's potting mixes – but it is rose thorns that often cause the wound/entry point and serve to introduce the infective fungal spores, hence the condition's common names of rose gardener's disease and rose thorn illness.

What happens next has as much to do with your personal immune response and any underlying condition (diabetes, etc.) as it does with any conforming pathology. For most, the disease manifests as a wound complication and does not progress beyond the skin, but for some it becomes a local lympho-cutaneous infection that develops a week or more (up to twelve days) after the thorn prick. At the wound site, papules or nodules (pimple to boil sized) will form and may ulcerate; this is the cutaneous part. But later more nodules may arise following along the proximal lymphatic route from the injury point – this is the lympho part – and your system is compromised. This can lead to complications such as disseminated sporotrichosis – where the infection spreads to joints and bones or into the central nervous system and the brain.

I should note that *Sporothrix schenckii* may be inhaled, as with any spore among your garden plants and soil, and if so a pulmonary infection can occur. This is a very rare occurrence and not considered as an occupational injury, while wound-infected

77

sporotrichosis is – particularly for gardeners, agricultural workers and vets (cats can carry it and they scratch too).

FIRST RESPONSE

The manifestation of the illness is slow, but if you are concerned after a thorn scratch or splinter, then clean the wound site with a strong antiseptic and take some supplements to boost your immune system. This may do the trick, but if infection develops and produces ulcerated boils or progresses to the lymphatic stage, then prescription antifungal medication will be required – often for several months. Complications may require hospitalisation.

GARDEN AID

Echinacea tea or echinacea cordial (see cordial concentrate recipe on page 79) will support your immune system to better fight the infection, but you will require a lymphatic herb to clear and calm the inflamed lymph nodes. Red clover flower and cleavers are excellent as lymphatic tonics: blend with strawberries for a lymphatic tonic smoothie, or to make up as a tincture – both can also be applied topically to infected nodes.

Top tip

How to remove thorns. Best practice is to grip any protrusion with tweezers and pull slowly. Follow with an antiseptic rinse and consider your current tetanus status. Embedded thorns can be treated as one would splinters, with a hot poultice or a drawing salve remedy (see page 172) to draw them out.

Rose Gardener's Draughts

Quick immune response booster

Make a really strong pot of echinacea tea – leaving four to five bags in the pot for 30 minutes minimum, and while the tea is hot stir in four tablespoons of honey and the juice of one lemon. Allow the mixture to cool, then decant into a tall glass and add a fizzy vitamin C tablet to quickly have a refreshing and immunity-revitalising beverage. Or have the drink as an iced tea. Take the mixture once a day for one month (with weekends off for best results – short bursts of treatment alternated with breaks make echinacea more effective).

Slower 'infection-busting' cordial concentrate

INGREDIENTS

½ cup grated ginger root

⅓ cup dried echinacea root, diced

⅓ cup elderberries *or* 1 cup blackberries

4 cups strong camomile tea – use several tea bags and let them brew for 30 minutes

Juice of a lemon, plus its grated zest

Juice of an orange, plus its grated zest

½ cup honey

1 fizzy zinc mineral tablet

Method

Mash the roots up in a mortar and pestle, add to a saucepan with the berries and three cups of camomile tea, and slowly bring to the boil. Add the juices and grated zests and allow to simmer for 20 minutes, adding extra tea if needed to maintain a good fluid level. Allow the mixture to rest for 20 minutes, then add the honey and the fizzy zinc capsule. Bring to the boil again stirring constantly and simmer for 10 minutes to reduce. Strain off the solids and decant the liquid into a bottle. It will keep in the refrigerator for up to five days. Use as a concentrated cordial by adding to chilled water (sparkling or still) for a daily or weekly boost.

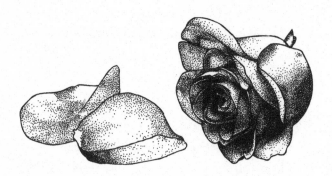

ACHES AND PAINS

Aches and pains are perhaps the most common complaints for gardeners – a result of the physicality of maintaining a garden. Some will have their origin in repetitive strains, some will be closer to an occupational injury, and others are just the wrong move at the wrong moment, when a muscle or tendon is stretched that bit too far.

In this section we shall explore some of the more frequent sites of aches and pains, looking at first responses that can lessen their potential to debilitate the gardener. Aid can be found from the kitchen as well as the garden (unless, of course, you keep a pineapple hothouse – which covers both) with a glass of anti-inflammatory pineapple juice to drink, or some chilli and turmeric paste to apply. Pineapple compresses have been employed for sprains, strains and skin infections in South American ethnobotany.

ACHILLES TENDON INJURIES

There are a range of complications and conditions that can impact upon the Achilles tendon – a tendon prone to overuse by active people such as joggers, ramblers, hill climbers and, of course, gardeners. The prime agent of injury is stepping up a gear in physical activity too quickly or without warming up/stretching first. In a less acute stage, prolonged activity and general wear and tear can be aggravated by flat feet and ill-fitting or non-ergonomic shoes.

TYPES OF INJURY

- Achilles tendon tears – sudden onset tears resulting in pain, inflammation and impaired movement.
- Achilles tendonitis – occurs when frequent activity gradually inflames the tendon, delivering pain, swelling and defined stiffness at the back of the heel.
- Achilles tendinosis – the gradual thickening of the tendon, often without any apparent inflammation, either through ageing or from overworking the tendon. It weakens the tissue and makes one prone to repetitive injury.
- Ruptures of the Achilles tendon often make an audible 'pop', followed by strong pain and noticeable swelling of the ankle and lower leg. This requires surgery to correct.

If left unchecked, a tendon injury can become a recurrent problem or lead to a more serious rupture and a period of in-capacitation followed by a period of physical therapy and hampered gardening. The symptoms of an increasing injury to the Achilles tendon are tenderness, swelling or general stiffness at the ankle/heel; a burning sensation in the back of the heel; mild to severe pain along the back of the foot and above the heel; ankle/heel and foot pain upon flexing or stretching the ankle or upon standing on tiptoe. If you hear a snap, crackle or pop, it's not your breakfast but a rupture. Similarly, if you have some difficulty in flexing your foot, or indeed pointing your toes, it indicates a more complete tear or rupture.

FIRST RESPONSE ⊕

PRICE: Protect, Rest, Ice, Compression (bandage wrap)

and Elevation – and if required augment with some over-the-counter pain relief. More serious tears and ruptures will require professional medical supervision and expertise, necessitating immobilisation casts and potential surgery to reattach the ruptured tendon.

GARDEN AID

Post-PRICE one may use herbs that flush blood into, and toxins out of, the affected site and are conducive to a speedy recovery. A mustard powder and yarrow leaf foot bath will fit the bill, or you can make a 1:2 ratio (herb to alcohol) arnica tincture or rustle up an instant 1:1 horse chestnut paste (see page 47) – both are effective for capillary stability, bruise resolution and pain relief. Passionflower tea (leaf infusion) contains apigenin – a nervine and antispasmodic agent for all types of neuralgia.

BACKACHE

We gardeners are prone to the odd bout of backache, which is only natural given the physicality of the hobby/occupation we enjoy. Sometimes it is just a mild strain that can be walked off or which dissipates within minutes. However, at other times it is a strain or overworking that requires a change of activity and some heat to remedy. The ache can signify a more pronounced injury (slipped discs, torn ligaments, etc.) that will require recuperation and the attention of a medical professional.

Lumbar/Lower back pain is certainly the commonest type of backache that gardeners suffer from. That region is the hinge of the majority of our gardening activities and as such is prone to experience overuse and strain, thus triggering tension and stiffness as a defence mechanism or warning sign. If unheeded or not noticed in the fervour of getting the last of the bulbs in, it slips easily over that line into soreness and then on to definite pain. The lumbar region is hinged by five vertebrae that act to support the weight of your upper body. That weight is added to any incorrect postural stance when strimming, pruning roses or digging, and it compounds strain when you bend awkwardly or lift incorrectly. Ergonomic posture is vital to avoid backache becoming a regular feature of your gardening activities.

Upper and middle back pain is rarer, or at least rarely to do with the action injuries (bending awkwardly or lifting incorrectly) that gardeners' actions might contribute towards. The vertebrae here, known as the thoracic vertebrae, are not required to move and flex like the lumbar vertebrae, and the ache, which can range from a dull stiffness to a sharp or burning sensation, is more likely to be the result of a pinched nerve or referred lung or rib pain. That said, poor task-posture can trigger upper and middle back pain, so when trimming the top of a hedge or carrying out a similar chore, try to keep your back as straight as possible, always balance your weight evenly on both feet and take frequent breaks.

First response ✚

Depending on the depth of pain, a rub to flush some blood into the muscle involved is ideal and a 'walk-off' may just do the trick. But if the area is inflamed and walking it off is not an option, then an ice pack will be required to reduce swelling and numb pain. Over-the-counter pain relief (aspirin, ibuprofen, etc.) are the norm.

Top tip

When applying an ice pack always wrap it in a towel or cloth – any kind of barrier to avoid direct skin contact – and never use it for more than 20 minutes at a time. Breaks of 30–45 minutes between icing treatments are advised. Cold therapy only works on day one, so if the pain or ache is still there the next day, using heat packs or counter-irritant salves can provide relief.

Garden aid

Many garden plants can be used as natural pain relief in tea and tincture form. Pain relief herbs include angelica, bay, birch, lavender, motherwort, peppermint, skullcap, St John's wort, valerian and, of course, willow bark (the original aspirin). Many over-the-counter creams and rubs for back pain contain methyl salicylates from the mint family, or use arnica, eucalyptus, rosemary or wintergreen.

Quick Salve for the Speedy Relief of Backache, Sciatica, Tired Limbs and Sore Muscles

Cayenne spice stimulates endorphin production when taken internally but also to a degree when absorbed through the skin. It is analgesic and anti-inflammatory.

Simply mix a teaspoon of cayenne pepper with a teaspoon of ground ginger, a teaspoon of dried mint (the latter two are also beneficial to pain relief and toxin flushing) with two tablespoons of vodka/brandy and a tablespoon of petroleum jelly or aqueous solution (or an alternative base of shea butter or coconut oil). I warm the mixing spoon in boiling water to help to slightly melt and blend all the ingredients, before mixing well and smearing over the painful site. The generated heat and pain-modifying properties offer relief, which is especially beneficial after initial cold therapy. You can boost the potency of this recipe by replacing the alcohol content with a tincture of analgesic herbs – try one, or a combination of, arnica, wintergreen and feverfew.

Muscle sprain/pulled muscle/ ligament injury

Muscle sprain is often referred to as a pulled muscle, but it is in fact a ligament injury. Sprains are painful (and debilitating), while strains are closer to an ache (and wear off). Ligaments are the tough straps – quite similar to elastic bands in action – that connect bone to bone and secure joints in place. A sprain results from the tearing of ligament fibres, sometimes partial, sometimes fully torn. The more intense the pain and the larger the swelling, the more likely it is to be a complete tear, which may necessitate surgery. Apart from the knee and ankle (common injury sites for gardeners), there are ligaments at every joint.

First response

Apply RICE – Rest, Ice, Compression (bandage wrap) and Elevation – with the 'rest' portion being for at least 48 hours. If no improvement is noted on day three after the injury, then visit a GP for evaluation. If the joint feels unstable or numb, medical assistance should be sought on the day of the injury. RICE is often complemented by heat packs or sprain plasters on days two and three.

Garden aid

A refreshing herbal tea fresh from the garden, with plants selected to improve blood flow to damaged structures, is the ticket. Make a blend of any three of the following: linden flowers, gingko leaves, hawthorn leaves, prickly ash bark and

87

yarrow flowers. All are excellent for encouraging peripheral circulation.

KITCHEN AID

With strong inflammation, the body's adrenal glands release the natural anti-inflammatory defence chemical cortisone. Turmeric improves the uptake and absorption of cortisone at sites of stress – include it in a topical compress or add to the quick relief salve on page 86. You can take it as part of your normal diet too – in your favourite curry, or mix it with your favourite butter or non-butter spread to give a zing to hot toast or a bling glaze to boiled potatoes.

Sprained Muscle Plaster

Both horsetail and comfrey have been part of herbal tissue repair remedies for centuries, as the silica content and some of their other phytochemicals help to build connective tissues. Both were taken internally up to recent times, but this remedy is for topical application.

INGREDIENTS

½ cup horsetail leaves and stems *or* 30 drops of tincture

½ cup chopped comfrey leaves and stems *or* 30 drops of tincture

½ cup chopped birch, willow or ash leaves *or* 2 crushed aspirin tablets

½ cup vinegar (any kind)

3 tablespoons grated ginger root

3 tablespoons mustard powder

1 tablespoon ground turmeric

Cornflour to thicken

Water to dilute

METHOD

Add 2 cups of water and all the ingredients except the cornflour to a saucepan and bring to the boil, then cover and rest the mixture away from the heat for 20 minutes. Stir well, or whisk with a hand blender. Finally thicken or dilute, as necessary, with cornflour or extra water. Leave it to sit for a minute or two, then once it is at a comfortable temperature apply to the sprained area, using a cling film 'bandage' to keep it in place if required. Leave on for half an hour before rinsing clean.

The quantity above should provide several applications over a two- to three-day period. If there is no improvement by then, the tear may be more serious and in need of medical intervention.

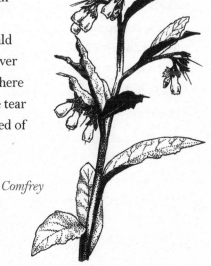

Comfrey

Muscle strain/aching muscles

Muscle strain is not as severe as muscle pull (sprain). It is not about torn or stretched ligaments but rather the dull ache of overworking a muscle. It is one of the most common gardening complaints. It can manifest in a stiffness and progress to a pain or heaviness in the affected limb or region of the muscle. The aim is first to cool the ache, then improve the blood flow to the area affected to detox the tissues and speed recovery. Do not work through the strain – you are not a footballer walking off a light cramp; that said we can steal a trick from sports medicine and learn to employ ice packs early, while maintaining the strained muscle in a stretched position.

First response ⊕

The priceless system of PRICE (protection, rest, ice, compression and elevation) is the first port of call, and later a flushing of the toxins that build up in overworked muscles will speed recovery. When it comes to the ice part, applying it 15–20 minutes in every hour while awake will both numb pain and reduce inflammation. The compression is simply a gently applied elastic bandage which, when combined with elevation, decreases swelling and forces the casualty to rest.

Garden aid

A delicious cup of yarrow and linden flower tea is both calming and improves blood supply to sore muscles, to naturally flush away the agents of ache – lactic acid, toxins, haematomas, etc. Gingko, rosemary, peony and ginger are all beneficial too.

KITCHEN AID

A simple kitchen cure is to add a dash of pain-relieving spice to your evening meal for a few days. I would opt for turmeric, ginger, cayenne or chilli. If you don't fancy a stir-fry or curry, try a teaspoon of any of these in a glass of juice; add a pinch of salt and you have hydration of the muscle at the same time.

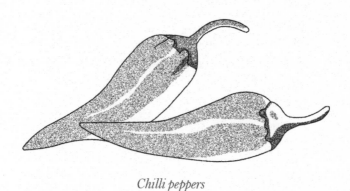

Chilli peppers

Sore Muscle Salve

Here is a stimulating and remedial salve for sore muscles, with warming herbs and analgesic and antispasmodic action.

INGREDIENTS

10 garden mint leaves

20 catmint leaves

1 sprig rosemary

1½ cups olive oil *or* alternative vegetable or nut carrier oil

20g pure beeswax

¼ cup grated ginger root

1 tablespoon cayenne pepper *or* 1 teaspoon mustard powder

10 cloves

Water to boil

YOU WILL ALSO NEED

A saucepan

Two glass Mason/Kilner jars or Pyrex bowls

A wooden spoon

Strainer/cheesecloth

A container to store the salve

METHOD

Wash your harvested herbs and dry them with a kitchen towel, then tear, crush or chop to help release their active principles.

Clean, peel and grate the ginger.

Place the herbs, cloves, ginger and pepper/mustard powder in a glass Mason/Kilner jar/Pyrex bowl and cover completely with the carrier oil. Seal the opening with cling film or kitchen parchment.

Bring a pan of water to the boil and turn off the heat, stand the herb-and-oil-filled glass jar or Pyrex bowl in the hot water and leave it to begin infusing. After 30 minutes, return the pan to the heat and simmer the water around the jar or bowl for a further 2 hours, adding water to the pan as evaporation occurs. After 2 hours, turn off the heat and allow the jar/bowl to sit in the hot water and continue infusing for a further 30 minutes, then strain off the herbs and other solids and decant the oil into the second jar/bowl.

Chip, shave or grate the beeswax into the hot infused oil and stir until it dissolves fully, adding gentle heat via a bain-marie if necessary. Allow to cool before decanting the mixture into your storage container, then leave to cool further and solidify before lidding and storing.

The average shelf life of a homemade salve is approximately a year from the date it was made (as long as your base oil was fresh to begin with) and stored in a cool location where it can remain semi-solid without continually re-melting and re-solidifying, thus spoiling.

Neck ache/Stiff neck

The biggest pain in the neck may be slugs this month, greenfly the next … and certainly those irritations can cause genuine tension headaches and allied neck pain. But the other stresses of the garden, physical stresses, are liable to get you in the neck at some point too. Most of your body muscles will relax completely when not actively being used, but the muscles of the neck are permanently tense in their work of supporting your head.

The average head weighs in at between 4.5kg and 9kg, set above seven small vertebrae and held in place by thirty-two complex muscles. Looking above or below your eye level for long periods, such as when pruning a tree or weeding between vegetable rows, can strain the neck's components to the point of later manifesting stiffness or tightness, or triggering a dull ache or even a sharp pain.

Neck pain can resolve itself in a matter of hours, or days at the most, but beyond the temporary stress-type sore neck, repetitive strain and wear and tear can impact on the gardener's cervical spine too. Anything more prolonged will be an indication of more chronic soft-tissue abnormalities, inflammatory disease or some cervical disk degeneration, medically termed spondylosis – all of which would necessitate medical supervision and guided treatments.

If pain is caused by a strain rather than an injury (which always means a trip to consult a medical professional), over-the-counter painkillers or herbal pain-relieving tea will also help.

94

First response ⊕

Our natural response is to rub tired, aching muscles, and the massaging action flushes blood in and toxins or lactic acid out, helping to speed recovery. But the application of a bag of frozen vegetables in a tea towel for 15 minutes at a time is excellent cold therapy and works to decrease inflammation in the neck faster than a rub.

Later, a little heat therapy – a quick, hot shower or resting for 10 minutes with a heat pack – will flush the site, easing stiffness and ache, and speed recovery. If the heat aggravates the soreness then more than likely you have an inflammatory condition and should return to the ice pack, use some natural anti-inflammatories and make an appointment for a medical investigation.

Garden aid

Harvest some natural herbs from the garden to make a cooling gel. Blend a handful of mint leaves and ten drops of rosemary or wintergreen essential oil with a dollop of coconut oil or carrier oil of your choice to make a cooling massage lotion.

Kitchen aid

Blend a small chilli pepper and ten drops of cypress essential oil with a dollop of coconut oil or carrier oil of your choice to make a warming and analgesic rub.

Infused Capsicum Rubbing Oil for Hot Therapy Treatment of Aches and Pains

Over-the-counter gels and creams for lower back pain characteristically include menthol, methylsalicylate and camphor from plant sources. They are often called counter-irritants or rubefacients as they create a warming or cooling sensation that on one level distracts your mind from the pain sensation, and on another heats or cools the sore muscle that is triggering the ache. They also increase blood flow to flush away toxins. Some, especially those featuring capsicum, may interfere more directly with the neural signals that transmit pain sensations to the brain and help to desensitise the area experiencing pain.

INGREDIENTS

250ml rapeseed oil (or carrier of choice)

3 tablespoons cayenne powder

3 tablespoons chilli flakes

A pan of boiling water

A glass jar with a tightly fitting lid

METHOD

Simply place the carrier oil in a jam jar or Mason/Kilner jar and add the dry ingredients. Put on the lid and sit the jar in the pan of boiling water. Simmer for 20 minutes and allow to cool fully. You may strain away the chilli flakes at this point, or leave to continue cold-infusing. Use as needed – the mixture stores for six months.

The oil may be warmed gently before every application if desired, but try it cold first to check for skin sensitivity to capsicum.

CUTS AND GRAZES

Cuts and grazes are common occurrences and there are different levels of injury, but the common denominators in treatment are to stop bleeding, clean the wound and protect it from infection. If bleeding is an issue, see pages 112–18, and also page 278 on assessing the need for stitches.

ABRASIONS: FIRST DEGREE/SCRAPE OR LIGHT GRAZE

Abrasions are perhaps the most common injuries from which gardeners suffer; they include those surface layer wounds that are often not noticed at the point of injury but may smart or sting later in the day – a scraped knuckle, a lightly skinned knee, a scratch along your arm from a thorn or a cane, an incident of friction between skin and wall or other abrading surface. Most abrasions will heal quickly and without scarring or complications, once they are cleaned and kept clean for a few days after the incident. They generally resolve within a week, but abrasions, like any laceration or wound, if not treated promptly and properly may become contaminated by dirt or dust particles and are then liable to septic infection as well as a spectrum of bacterial infections.

A first-degree abrasion involves superficial damage to the epidermal layer of skin; bleeding is minimal, if present at all.

FIRST RESPONSE ⊕

Wash the site with soapy water to remove any debris and follow up with an antiseptic wipe, liquid dab, or iodine or ointment application. Slight stinging may arise in the process of cleaning and sterilising.

GARDEN AID

The garden offers an array of natural antiseptics that can quickly be used. A rub of crushed or torn calendula petals or a smear of aloe vera gel will clean and seal the wound from potential secondary infection.

If the abrasion was from a doubtful surface or source, then an infusion of thyme is an excellent wound healer with instant antiseptic and anti-microbial properties. The trick is in its thymol content, which is similar in anti-microbial potential to carbolic acid and as effective as iodine or phenol-based antiseptics.

Thyme Antiseptic Rinse

Thyme infusions and oil of thyme have an ancient lineage in healing, going back to the Egyptians and the origins of medicinal botany. Before the discovery of antibiotics, doctors once soaked bandages in thyme to disinfect the cloth, kill germs on the surface of wounds and help activate healing. The active antibiotic principle in thyme – thymol – is considered to be twenty-five times as effective as phenol (the active ingredient in most over-the-counter antiseptics).

INGREDIENTS

1 bunch thyme (several sprigs) *or* 2 tablespoons of the dried herb

1 cup water

METHOD

As you would make a herbal tea, garden-grown thyme can simply be harvested, torn or crushed to open a pathway to the volatile oils and phytochemicals within, then added to boiling water and steeped for a few minutes, before straining and cooling to yield a soothing wound rinse.

This is intended for immediate use but can be stored in the refrigerator for several days. It is suitable also as a remedy for coughs, sore throats, colds and flu, and headaches in the form of a herbal tea. Or can be applied to cuts, infected wounds, yeast infections and athlete's foot.

Top tip

Adding some lavender or rosemary herb to the mix will boost its disinfectant properties.

Aromatic skin-graze rinse

Use the same ingredients and method as for the thyme rinse, but with equal quantities of thyme and bee balm (which also contains thymol) and a few rose petals, to tone skin and enhance the all-round aroma.

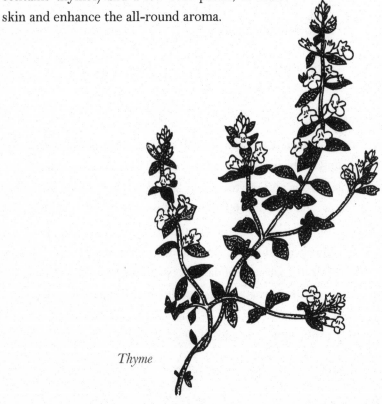

Thyme

100

ABRASIONS: SECOND DEGREE/ GRAZES WITH BLOOD SPOTTING

A second-degree abrasion, regarded more often as a scrape or graze, involves both the epidermis as well as the dermis layers of skin and so may bleed slightly.

FIRST RESPONSE

Similar to that of a first-degree abrasion: clean the wound and apply preventative antiseptic.

GARDEN AID

Wash the abrasion with lukewarm homemade thyme or camomile tea to disinfect the wound, pat dry with a clean cloth and seal the wound site with a coat of petroleum jelly (with no sting, this is a great option for kids), or you could use honey to cover and protect the wound. With the use of petroleum jelly it is safe to re-enter the garden, but honey may attract insects. However, both act to soothe and keep the wound moisturised – which is key to a speedy recovery.

Top tip

Spit clean the wound. Saliva contains several antimicrobial and disinfectant agents as well as promoting wound healing and skin regeneration – simply spit on and rub in.

Avocado Graze Glaze

For second-degree abrasions and sundry grazes where inflammation occurs, or for larger surface abrasions, a poultice of pulped avocado flesh is sublime. The oil is so close to our skin's natural oil that it has been employed as a nourishing treatment for centuries. Its high content of skin- and wound-healing vitamins, including potent quantities of vitamins E, A and C, is what makes its regenerative powers so beneficial to cuts, scrapes, grazes and scratches.

INGREDIENTS

1 avocado, with stone removed

A few teaspoons oatmeal (optional)

You will also need a blender or a sturdy potato masher

METHOD

Depending on the ripeness of the avocado, scoop and mash the flesh or slice and blitz it to the consistency of a paste. It is recommended to apply an avocado poultice or pulp paste to the affected site for three consecutive days. You can add oatmeal to thicken the paste if needed. To hold it on awkwardly positioned wounds, you can apply the paste and cover it with a bandage. For most types of second-degree abrasions and grazes, just a smear will suffice. Avocado pulp paste will keep in the fridge for the best part of a week.

Note: The fruit pulp of avocado with its broad array of anti-inflammatory carotenoids helps to reduce the pain, irritation and inflammation associated with second-degree abrasions. But it is known also to hasten the process of healing in all skin conditions and can be used as a recovery treatment where skin requires some TLC (including scars, rashes and burns).

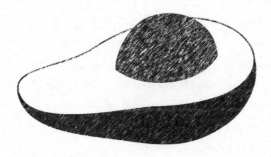

Avocado

ABRASIONS: THIRD DEGREE/AVULSION INJURY

A third-degree abrasion, also known as an avulsion injury, involves more tear than wear and takes damage further into the subcutaneous layer of skin. There are levels of damage, and a third-degree injury on a finger or hand/knee, while uncomfortable and impeding to some garden chores, is easily remedied and heals within weeks. Larger or deeper avulsions can become complicated, though, and need more healing time, medication and sometimes grafts and so on.

Gardeners can suffer a third-degree abrasion from a fall, an encounter with a rough-faced wall or the odd war wound caused when removing branches, old posts or stubborn ivy, etc. A layer of thumb can be scraped away with nearly half of the garden chores we do. A more serious avulsion injury, such as where a falling branch or felled tree strips away a section of flesh, will require medical treatment – call for help and an ambulance. Shock can quickly become a factor with such traumas too.

FIRST RESPONSE

Tradition dictates 'debriding' or cleaning the wound site and the application of a mild antiseptic, often hydrogen peroxide (popular in commercial first aid kits), before wound dressing. However, it has recently been found that the use of hydrogen peroxide may in fact impair the natural automatic process of wound healing.

With third-degree wound dressing there are three phases – first, to bandage for a few days with daily changes of the dressing; then, as the wound begins to heal, move to keeping it covered during the day and open to the air at night. Finally, when the injured area has dried up and scabbed over, bandages can be left off and care changed to using a soothing antiseptic cream. In all stages, watch out for any spreading redness or discoloration in or around the wound site, any swelling or increase in pain, discharge of pus or any odour – all of these indicate infection and the need for medical supervision. With more serious abrasions (over a large or deep area, or caused by suspected contaminated material – for example, an old fencing panel, where wooden splinters and insect dander may also be embedded in the wound) tetanus immunisation status becomes relevant. See 'tetanus' on pages 178–9.

GARDEN AID

While severe avulsions are best checked over and cleaned by a medical professional, a rinse with an antiseptic tea is beneficial to disinfect the wound immediately and to promote faster healing. Thyme, lavender, camomile or rosemary will all serve this purpose. Assess whether stitches may be needed, or further professional assistance; if not, then a clean dressing or honey plaster will render the wound safe and allow the natural processes to begin. A wash of infused nasturtium flowers and leaves is antibiotic. The fruits of forsythia are similarly used in traditional Chinese medicine as an anti-infective.

Cuts/lacerations

Nicks and cuts are among the most common types of gardening injury, along with bumps, grazes and backache. Anything bleeding or with opened skin is termed a 'cut' – whether it is a cut, slice or tear injury. In fact, medically or descriptively, there are several types of cut, most often categorised by depth or type of wound, and the two that concern gardeners the most are incised and lacerated cuts.

An *incised* cut is a sharper or more surgical wound than a laceration – it is commonly caused by a sharp metal edge, broken glass or a mishap with a Stanley knife or craft blade, etc. It can even be the dreaded paper cut from a seed packet.

A *lacerated* cut is a little rougher around the edges, more of a rip than of surgical precision – the sort of cut you could get from a pruning saw or other sharp-edged object.

First response ✚

If the cut is bleeding, stop the bleeding with simple pressure; if it is not bleeding, wash the wound, then apply antiseptic and an adhesive plaster or other dressing to prevent secondary infection. Nothing more is needed unless the cut was made by a rusty implement (see 'tetanus' on pages 178–9) or contaminated by animal waste (see 'zoonoses' on pages 20–1) or other wound pollutants – in these cases a medical check-up and antibiotics may be required.

Most gardeners' cuts are superficial and heal in a matter of days, but they must be kept clean and a wary eye kept for signs of infection (redness, swelling, oozing). Only occasionally might they need preventive treatment for a higher risk of infection. Deep or extensive cuts, or cuts that may have venous or arterial bleeds, are medical emergencies and need immediate attention.

For any injury with spurting blood, stop the bleeding by applying direct pressure to the wound: use your hand or an improvised dressing. It may seem counter-intuitive, but sit the injured person down and get them to relax as resting reduces the risk of fainting as well as helping to control the bleeding. This, combined with a calm sense of purpose, means the patient's heart doesn't have to pump at panic strength.

GARDEN AID

Yarrow staunches blood – use a compress of the fresh herb – and makes an excellent antiseptic. It is also a brilliant wound cleaner when mixed with a strained thyme infusion. Bistort is strongly astringent – both the leaves and the root – with a long history in the treatment of internal and external bleeding. A topically applied comfrey root paste, leaf compress or juice contains allantoin, which stimulates cell division, thus speeding the healing process. A rub of fresh calendula flowers or a homemade calendula salve (see page 108, the 'cut and paste' recipe) stimulates a faster healing response too. Botanical antiseptics you could use in a salve or tincture include chickweed, echinacea, elderflower, goldenseal, lavender, thyme and sage.

Three Recipes for Sealing and Soothing Cuts

Cut and paste recipe

To a mortar and pestle add a finger-length of cleaned root of comfrey or two finely chopped comfrey leaves; five fresh calendula flower heads or a handful of camomile flowers; a tablespoon of clove oil or a teaspoon of ground clove spice; and a tablespoon of olive oil. Mash the ingredients to a paste and apply to the cut. The salve can be stored in the fridge for five days.

Cut and glue recipe

Warm a dollop (around 2 heaped tablespoons) of petroleum jelly or coconut oil in a bain-marie and add a half teaspoon each of ground cloves, ground cinnamon and cayenne pepper. Stir well and let the mixture cool to a stiff consistency. The mixture will store conveniently in a bathroom cabinet for several months. Use as required to seal cuts and wounds – this has active antiseptic and antibiotic properties.

Cut and super glue recipe

No superglue needed – that was developed for military or combat first aid, but our method is less sticky. Prepare a mixture as for the 'cut and glue' recipe above, but before the mixture sets break into it a capsule of vitamin E plus 10 drops of lavender essential oil and 10 drops of tea tree essential oil. Stir well and leave to set. This salve will store for several months in your first aid kit, or even on a shelf in the shed. Use as required to seal cuts and wounds requiring stronger active antiseptic and antibiotic properties.

Honey Plaster

This is a simple recipe, requiring only honey, gauze and a bandage.

METHOD

Just slather the honey over the pre-cleaned wound, lay a layer of gauze over it and bandage the wound. Change the dressing twice daily until the injury has healed sufficiently to expose to the air.

Scar tissue treatment

Essential oil of angelica is an excellent healer of wounds and scars – it can be added to honey plasters or, if specifically for old scar tissue, can be used in rubbing blends with avocado oil or coconut oil.

Antiseptic Herbal Tincture

INGREDIENTS

2 tablespoons basil leaves, chopped

2 tablespoons bergamot leaves/flowers, chopped

3 tablespoons thyme leaves/flowers, chopped

3 tablespoons peppermint leaves, chopped

2 sprigs lavender

2 sprigs rosemary

200ml vodka *or* grain spirit

METHOD

Add all the herb ingredients to the vodka/spirit and leave the mixture in a Mason/Kilner-type glass jar on a sunny window sill for two weeks. Then strain away the herbs and store the liquid in an airtight dark glass bottle in a dry cupboard. The mixture will store for one year. Use when needed as an antiseptic wash or a dabbing liquid.

Essential Antiseptic Ointment

A quickly produced healing ointment based on the antiseptic properties of four essential oils – eucalyptus (anti-inflammatory, antiseptic and antibacterial), lavender (analgesic, antibiotic, anti-fungal and antibacterial), tea tree oil (antibiotic, anti-fungal and antibacterial) and thyme (antibiotic, antiseptic, anti-fungal and antibacterial).

INGREDIENTS

20g pure beeswax

1 cup almond or other carrier oil of choice

2 heaped tablespoons cocoa butter *or* shea butter

20 drops eucalyptus essential oil

20 drops lavender essential oil

20 drops tea tree essential oil

20 drops thyme essential oil

METHOD

Grate the beeswax into a Pyrex bowl and add the carrier oil and vegetable butter. Then, using a bain-marie, heat and melt them together. Remove from the heat and add the essential oils. Stir well with a chopstick or the handle of a wooden spoon. Pour the mixture into a suitable container – a sterilised jar or recycled tins. Allow to cool and set naturally. Store in a cool, dark place and use as needed.

This ointment will keep for several years but I like to make it fresh annually. Apart from blisters, cuts and minor wounds, it is great for chapped hands, tired feet and 'boot foot' too – so a surplus is never around for long.

BLEEDING AND WOUNDS

Beyond little nicks and scrapes, some injuries will require at least an understanding of the control of bleeding as well as of wound management. Many can be addressed with techniques covered in the core skills section of this book and the application of homemade solutions, but professional medical advice is advised for any open wound.

MINOR BLEEDING

Cuts, scrapes, nicks and avulsion wounds – whether caused by a tool mishap, a shard of glass in the soil, a nail in a trellis or whatever – can all be deep enough to trigger a run of blood. When it comes to a minor bleed (non-spurting, slow or minimal flow) the main aim is to stop it, prevent further loss of blood and minimise any potential infection.

FIRST RESPONSE ⊕

Applying pressure to stem blood loss will be called for, but the first step is to check that there is nothing embedded in the wound site (glass, splinter, etc.) before applying any dressing or pressure.

If the wound does not have an embedded object, you will need to apply and maintain a firm (but not squeezing) pressure to the wound, using a clean pad or gauze beneath your hand. If possible, cup the wound with your palm and hold for 10 minutes before proceeding to clean and dress the wound site.

If the wound is on a limb (without other damage or fracture), then raising it will decrease the blood flow and speed clotting.

If the wound has an embedded object do not press down on the object but instead press firmly on both sides of the object to stem the flow of blood. Build up padding around the sides to avoid putting pressure on the object itself when you bandage the wound to hold back sustained blood loss. Get to a GP or hospital to have the embedded object removed professionally, in case it is piercing or close to nicking a major blood vessel. If the wound is large or in a precarious place (neck, groin, major artery sites), then call emergency services to provide assistance and transport.

GARDEN AID

The leaves of many garden plants and common weeds are able to stop blood flow/trigger clotting, including bistort, cranesbill geranium, lady's mantle, *Vinca* species, shepherd's purse and, of course, yarrow. Use as a compress. Quick tinctures can also be made (with any single herb or a combination of these herbs in a 1:2 ratio of herbal content to a vodka or brandy base) and used on cotton pads as swabs.

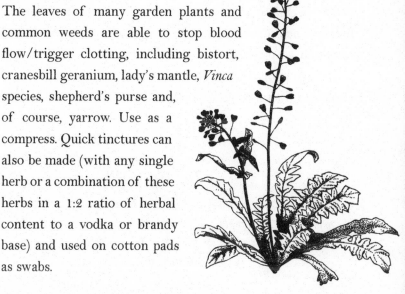

Shepherd's purse

113

MAJOR BLEEDING

Major bleeding is a medical emergency – always alert the emergency services. The flow of blood from a wound depends on which type of blood vessel has been damaged – arterial blood loss is bright red in colour as it spurts out (with each beat of the heart), but will darken when it meets the air. Venous bleeding is already dark and steady in flow.

When it comes to a major bleed of either sort, the main aim is to stop it, then stabilise the wound to prevent further loss of blood and proceed to minimise the effects of shock and casualty distress.

FIRST RESPONSE ✚

Call for help and for the emergency services. With a dressing or a clean cloth if possible, apply direct pressure to the wound, firm but not squeezing – squeezing might pinch the wound open and keep the blood flowing. Use a firm grip and hold to maintain pressure. If it is a limb wound and there is no suspected fracture, elevate the wound site above the level of the heart.

> ### *Top tip*
>
> *If dressings become soaked with blood, add more layers over them rather than replacing them with a clean dressing, as the less a bleeding wound is disturbed, the quicker it will begin clotting.*

114

Failure to control bleeding with a dressing, pressure and elevation necessitates a step up to pressure point control at the nearest point above the cut to stop or slow blood flow to the wound long enough for natural clotting to occur and to stem further blood loss. Pressure to these points should only be applied in increments – for no more than 10 minutes at a time. If bleeding continues after the first pressure period, repeat the pressure. If bleeding is not lessened during the pressure period, then the final procedure is to apply a pressure bandage over the wound. Wrap the wound site well with firm pressure but not so much as to constrict circulation to the extremities – check the pulse points to make sure and watch for fingertips or toes turning blue.

NOSEBLEED

From stepping on a rake, to high blood pressure, to dry air or a strong sneeze, the gardener can easily encounter a nosebleed. There are so many tiny blood vessels in the lining of the nose that bleeds can look profuse and dramatic, but it's not life-threatening and these ruptured capillaries will clot within several minutes (although this can take up to 20 minutes) and heal themselves completely in a few days. If it was a rake or other bump that caused the nosebleed, do not take aspirin or other blood-thinning pain relief, even after clots form.

FIRST RESPONSE

The nosebleed sufferer should sit or stand upright, leaning forward slightly to prevent swallowing blood and causing irritation to the throat or stomach. Upright and forward also reduces the blood pressure in the veins of the nose and facilitates clotting. Place the thumb and forefinger on each side of the nostrils and pinch them closed. Hold firmly for 10 minutes (clots take time) without releasing – the casualty should breathe through the mouth. After 10 minutes, slowly release the nostrils and check to see if the bleeding has ceased (do not prod about, pick at or clean clotted blood or blow the nose). If the bleeding has not stopped, then pinch again for a second 10-minute period, but if after that time there is still blood loss it is time to head for a GP or the emergency room.

GARDEN AID

A nose plug of yarrow can staunch blood flow. If you suffer regular nosebleeds you need to grow/eat more leafy vegetables, as their vitamin C, vitamin K and bioflavonoid content helps to strengthen any capillary fragility. Recurring bleeds could suggest an underlying condition, so seek medical advice.

KITCHEN AID

Vinegar can gently cauterise the capillary of the inner nose, so rather than using rolled-up plugs of damp tissue or folded plant leaves, try a vinegar-dipped cotton pad plug.

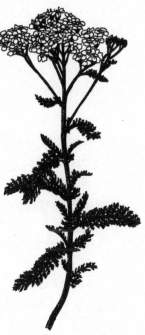

Yarrow

Minor Bleed Seal

All these ingredients are astringent and styptic, thus will tighten wounds and help to stop bleeding.

INGREDIENTS

2 heaped tablespoons shepherd's purse, chopped

1 heaped tablespoon fresh calendula petals

1 heaped tablespoon fresh yarrow flower heads

2 heaped tablespoons petroleum jelly *or* zinc ointment

20 drops geranium essential oil

METHOD

In a mortar and pestle, mash the shepherd's purse, fresh calendula petals and yarrow flower heads to a paste. Warm the petroleum jelly or zinc ointment and add to the herb paste with the geranium essential oil. Allow to set. This mixture stores for several months. Use as required to seal cuts and wounds.

Wounds

A 'wound' covers a multitude of different injuries, but it is generally accepted as a physical injury where the skin is cut, torn, pierced, punctured or otherwise broken. There is a universally recognised system of classification of wounds – using location of wound, wound depth, complexity of wound, wound age, origin of wound – all of which are needed to assess the seriousness of the situation and method of treatment, and are helpful to emergency services when making a distress call or seeking assistance.

If bleeding is profuse, the wound is extensive or you suspect organ or arterial damage, call the emergency services immediately. If it is a minor wound, but you suspect contamination or tetanus infection, seek professional medical treatment the same day. Of course, we can also have severed limbs from a chainsaw accident, and even crash injuries with ride-on lawnmowers, etc., and the cause or origin of the accident will help ambulance services to understand the severity of the situation and the needs of the casualty while en route to hospital.

There are also 'secondary wounds' originating from an underlying condition or primary disease which are rarely a complication of gardening, but some of the remedies and first responses would overlap – e.g. ulcerated chilblains and diabetic ulcers (but note the latter requires definitive medical supervision to avoid complications and serious consequences) and they could benefit from any treatment procedure or remedy listed in this book under abrasions.

119

CLASSIFICATION OF WOUNDS

Defining a wound is helpful to the 999/112 operator and to the emergency services en route.

1. Location of wound – where is it?
2. Wound depth.
    (a) Superficial – involves just the epidermis and the upper dermis.
    (b) Partial depth – comprises skin loss up to the lower dermis region.
    (c) Full depth – encompasses skin and subcutaneous tissue.
    (d) Deep – penetration into tissue, muscle, natural cavities or an organ.

3. Complexity of wound – what kind is it?
    (a) Simple wound – affects just one organ or tissue section.
    (b) Combined wound – implicates multiple organs and/or multiple tissues.

4. Age of wound.
    (a) Fresh – anywhere from 0–8 hours from the time of injury.
    (b) Old – longer than 8 hours from the time of initial injury.

5. Origin of wound – how it happened.
    (a) Superficial – a fall abrasion; scrape from a rough surface; scratching of an itch, etc.
    (b) Contused – injuries to tissue beneath the skin's surface, bruises and the like.

(c) Lacerated – rip cut by secateurs, scissors, pruning knife, saw or other sharp-edged object.

(d) Incised – a sharp or more surgical wound than a laceration – often caused by metal edges, broken glass, Stanley knife or craft blade, etc.

(e) Stab – a pointed tool.

(f) Punctured – nail gun or stepping on penetrating tool or nail.

(g) Impaled – falling onto a tool or sharp object.

(h) Crush – a pot or heavy weight falling on toe or body part, a felled tree incident, a heavy blow from a mis-aimed sledgehammer, etc.

(i) Bite – animal, spider, insect, snake.

(j) Burn – thermal, chemical, electric.

(k) Any other information you can give.

BURNS

There are quite a few ways to achieve/receive a burn in a gardening context (see below) and it can be confusing when burns are listed as minor, major, degree and type – so in an attempt to clarify, let's look at categories before types.

UNDERSTANDING CATEGORIES

The severity of a burn in first aid and medical terms really depends on its size, depth and location. Burns are considered most severe when located on the face, hands, feet, neck, groin and genitals, not just from a disfiguring point of view, but because these are regions where major blood vessels and limbic channels are located. Burns can be combined with other injuries – inhalation of smoke, electrocution, chemical poisoning, etc. Burns result in pain and potential infection, but of immediate concern is their potential to cause shock. Most garden burns are minor but, between autumn leaf bonfires, petrol mowers and strong caustic chemicals in the shed, an understanding of all types is useful.

There are several categories of burn (ranked by degrees or thickness) and many types (flame, scald, chemical, etc.), but all burns, no matter how deep/extensive or how they were acquired, are susceptible to tetanus (see pages 178–9) and will need medical follow-up beyond your first response.

Minor burns pertain to burns of a first degree nature, and of a second degree that are less than 7.5cm in diameter, e.g. a spill of a hot cup of tea, a brush against a hot iron, etc. and are not regarded as a medical emergency.

Major burns include second degree burns larger than the span of your hand or, if on the face or hands, larger than 7.5cm in diameter, and third degree (full thickness) burns of any dimension will require medical assistance.

Sunflower and Honey Ointment

A soothing ointment for wounds and cuts, post-burns and general skin repair.

Sunflower oil is a common ingredient found in kitchens, but, apart from its use for frying and salad dressings, it is one of those foodstuffs packed with vitamin E and so lends itself well to healing blends for skin conditions. In this treatment it is both part of the delivery method and an active agent in repairing damaged skin.

I give it a twist by infusing the oil with sunflower petals and other healing members of the sunflower family – Asteraceae/Compositae.

Goldenrod is a member of the sunflower family and its botanical name Solidago means 'to make whole'. Yarrow – the great wound healer – is also a member, as are the disinfectant Tagetes, the anti-inflammatory pot marigold/calendula (the oil of which increases collagen production, so helping to prevent or lessen the formation of scar tissue) and the antiseptic (but also anticoagulant – so select for certain wounds only) helichrysum. Pick and mix your own favourites. Allow to infuse for a minimum of two weeks.

INGREDIENTS

25g pure beeswax

100ml sunflower oil (infused or culinary)

100g honey

METHOD

Using a bain-marie, melt the beeswax in a few tablespoons of the oil, then add the rest of the oil and the honey and stir well together. Allow the mixture to cool. Store in a sealable jar in a kitchen cupboard, workbench drawer or medicine cabinet. Apply as needed to keep wounds moist and promote healing, taking advantage of the active parts of the skin-regenerating oil and the honey's power to prevent bacterial growth. Beeswax is also germicidal.

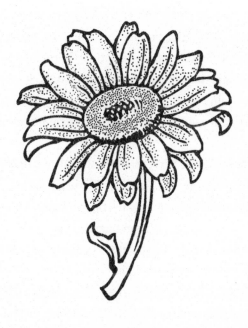

A Sunflower

DEGREES OF BURNS

FIRST RESPONSE TO A FIRST DEGREE BURN

First degree burns, also known as *superficial thickness burns,* are on the surface, where only the outer layer of skin is affected. They are painful but do not cause much more than redness and inflammation.

Flush the burn site with cool running water for at least 10 minutes, then apply moist dressings and bandage loosely to protect from secondary infection. If this degree of burn involves a substantial portion of the hands, feet, face, groin or a major joint, then it may be considered to be in the second degree category and likely to need medical intervention.

FIRST RESPONSE TO A MINOR SECOND DEGREE BURN

Second degree burns, also known as *partial thickness burns,* are more substantial – often in scale, but primarily in depth, where the first layer of skin has been burned through and the second layer compromised. Blistering regularly accompanies the redness and inflammation. Pain can be severe. (Technically, as noted earlier, if a second degree burn is less than 7.5 centimetres in diameter it is often treated as a minor burn – provided it does not affect hands, feet, face, groin or a major joint.)

Cool the burn and retard swelling by running it under cool water for about 10 minutes or until the pain reduces on contact with the air. Apply cling film or sterile gauze as a protective cover to the wound, but avoid fluffy cotton wool or lint. Wounds will be re-dressed in the emergency room or hospital, but if they are minor and suitable for home treatment, then remember to refresh the dressings daily.

FIRST RESPONSE TO A MAJOR SECOND DEGREE BURN

Skip the water flushing because of the potential for causing shock, and move to the application of dressings and a loose bandage or cling film wrap to protect the wound from contamination en route to hospital or while awaiting the ambulance.

FIRST RESPONSE TO A THIRD DEGREE BURN

Third degree burns, also known as *full thickness burns*, compromise all layers of the skin and generally cause permanent tissue damage. Damaged areas may be charred black or appear dry and white. In extreme circumstances fat, muscle and even bone may be affected. The casualty might not feel pain at the burn sites because of nerve damage.

Call for help and an ambulance, extinguish flames, do not remove burnt clothing. Check vital signs and begin CPR if required – otherwise calm the casualty with reassurance and cover the burn area with a moist bandage or damp cloths such as tea towels. Do not immerse the casualty in cold water as a sudden body temperature drop can speed the onset of shock. If possible, elevate the burnt body part while awaiting the emergency services. The casualty may go into shock or experience respiratory difficulty – if either of these happens, stay calm and place the casualty into a beneficial recovery position (see pages 260–1) until an ambulance or other emergency service arrives.

127

Types of burns

There are several different types of burns. The most common are *thermal burns*, caused by the dry heat of a flame, such as a garden bonfire, or the dry heat of a hot object, such as a garden incinerator, a barbecue grill, etc. Other common burns are *wet heat scalds* caused by steam or when weed killing with boiling water, or even the spilling of a hot cup of coffee.

But there are also *chemical*, *electrical* and *friction burns* – wearing leathers while gardening is not advised, but a mishap with a rope or other rasping surface happens all too easily. And, of course, burns to the skin from *solar radiation/sunburn* are very common in gardeners.

First response for all burns

TAKE CARE NOT TO ENDANGER YOURSELF

- Stop the burning process: if you are on fire don't run in a panic – stop, drop and roll or smother the flames with a jacket/blanket; if it is a chemical burn, then flush the chemical off the skin, remove contaminated clothes (unless they are adhering to the skin); if it is an electrical burn, turn off the electricity supply; if a scald or burn from a flame, run the scalded/burnt body part under a tap or the water from a running hose to halt the blister swell, etc.

- Cool the burning sensation – both to retard inflammation and numb pain. Begin with cool or lukewarm water, flushing for 10–15-minute intervals, but avoid direct contact with ice or iced water as this may be too cold and can trigger shock. Also, do not use antiseptic creams or greasy substances at this stage as they can slow cooling and contaminate wound visibility for paramedics.

- Protect the burn wound from further damage: cover the burn with cling film (strips rather than bandaging) or a moist, non-lint dressing.

- Protect the casualty from shock – a comfortable position and reassurance while waiting for the emergency services can help to slow the onset of both emotional and circulatory shock. Counter-intuitive as it may seem, a blanket or jacket over the shoulders or legs of a casualty can help him or her to relax and prevent shock, but do not cover the burnt area with extra layers.

OTHER ADVICE

- For anything above a minor burn or scald, call the emergency services at the first opportunity.

- If there is any fire or power line involvement, etc., call the emergency services – both fire and ambulance.

- If possible, remove rings or jewellery at the burn location before inflammation begins, but do not remove anything that is clearly stuck to burnt skin.

- When burnt by a garden or household chemical, if possible bag up its container to give to the paramedics or note the brand and active ingredient's name for hospital treatment and records.

Garden Aid

Major burns require medical intervention, but for first degree and minor burns aloe vera is an instant wound cooler. The sap is 96 per cent water and the other 4 per cent comprises active ingredients that nourish damaged skin, including amino acids and enzymes very beneficial to burns. The bruised leaves of acanthus have long been used in poultices to soothe burns and dress scalds. Plantain juice is cooling and antibacterial, and comfrey juice stimulates new skin formation. The infused leaves of lungwort destroy necrotic tissue and promote new skin formation. Goldenrod rinses will speed healing. Bistort (leaves and root) is strongly astringent, with a long history in the treatment of internal and external bleeding, but it is also useful, with thyme, to make a rinse for burns and wounds. Spit poultices also work well with minor garden burns.

Kitchen Aid

Cut some kitchen cling film into strips or patches, moisten and apply to the injured area as cling film dressings. Do not wrap as a bandage, simply lay on in layers.

Burn Recovery Gel

Aloe sap by itself is remedial to burns, but with the addition of some extra garden supplies a potent recovery gel to diminish scarring and promote skin health is easily made.

METHOD

Take three parts of aloe vera sap blended with one part of witch hazel extract and squeeze or press out the juice of comfrey, plantain and chickweed – a teaspoon of each to the three parts of aloe. Apply to non-raw or non-weeping wounds to soothe the damaged skin and bolster new skin formation.

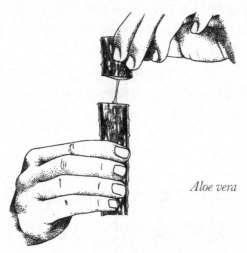

Aloe vera

Skin Tonic

METHOD

To 200ml of tonic water add ¼ cup of aloe vera sap and a crushed zinc tablet and shake well. Use as a tonic wash or spritz. Allow to dry naturally on the skin. Use several times daily during recovery – it can help to minimise scarring – unless wounds are bandaged or already treated with medicated gel. Post-bandaging, you can wash regularly in the solution.

Replenishing Skin Lotion

METHOD

Blend 200ml of witch hazel extract with the flesh of one avocado, a tablespoon of shea or cocoa butter and a tablespoon of honey. Apply as needed to boost your skin's natural regenerative powers. Can be part of your daily or weekly beauty regime or as a supplement when recovering from burns as a daily cleanse for the first few months post-injury. The mixture stores well for several months.

Peony burn recovery preparations – decoctions of dried root and tisanes of flowers

The first thing to note is that there are quite a few types of peony – some types predominate in Western herbals and others in traditional Chinese medicine – so I will use their

Latin names here to be more specific in terms of identification, purchase and usage.

Chinese peony, sold as *Paeonia lactiflora* in most garden centres, has a several-thousand-year history as a nervine, tonic and antispasmodic via a root soup, but a decoction of the roots is also analgesic, anodyne, antibacterial, antiseptic and anti-inflammatory, and so yields good advantage to burn recovery. Include in the diet during the first few weeks of recovery. If you cannot bear to dig up the roots of a garden favourite, visit your local Chinese herbalist for the dried root sold as bai shao (white peony) or chi shao (red peony) – both are excellent.

The other garden centre staple, *Paeonia suffruticosa*, is used in a similar manner and as an antibiotic. While not always available in mainstream garden centres, *Paeonia officinalis* also has all these qualities and in Western herbalism is prized as a sedative and pain easer – *officinalis* flowers

Peony

are used in infusions and tincture form for varicose veins and capillary health – the latter function is an ally to skin health and therefore also to burn recovery. Online and mail order *officinalis* seeds are easy to source.

CHEMICAL CONTACT

Even organic gardeners might have an old container of chemicals at the back of the shed, not to mention the array of household products with a chemical makeup. From bleach to fertiliser to lawnmower petrol, the garden can be a danger zone.

FIRST RESPONSE ✚

There are several procedural steps, but do note the name of the chemical involved and call poisons control in your local area for assistance (the emergency response operator will put you through) for swallowed rather than just skin contact chemicals. In some instances the chemicals may require induced vomiting to rid them from the system quickly, but with others this is the last thing you want to do; equally, some chemicals are best diluted internally with milk or water and others are not. There are so many garden chemicals and so many changes to product ingredients yearly that a list here would be redundant next week – EMS will advise on the latest protocol for the brand/chemical swallowed. Be it swallowed or surface contact, if possible, bag up the chemical container to give to the paramedics.

Decontaminate the casualty (remove chemical-soaked clothes, dilute chemicals on the skin with water if possible), get him or her into the fresh air, stabilise and reassure, and address any secondary wounds.

> ## *Top tip*
>
> *If you are dealing with a casualty rather than yourself, be sure to protect yourself from exposure to the chemical while administering first aid – wear gloves, a damp bandana around the mouth, etc.*

- *Pesticide and herbicide poisoning* – another good reason to go organic, as most garden chemicals – be they organophosphates, organochlorines, phenoxy herbicides, pyrethrins/pyrethroids, anticoagulant rodenticides, carbamates, or hypochlorite disinfectants – are serious toxins that require immediate medical attention. Worse still, pesticide and herbicide poisoning is one of the most common poisonings to happen within the garden. Seek protocol advice from EMS on the poison encountered while waiting for the ambulance.

- *Spill/splash/skin contact* – quickly rinse then wash the contaminated area with soap and water, but avoid harsh scrubbing which will only enhance pesticide absorption. If chemical burns of the skin have occurred, cover the wound area with a loose dressing and seek professional medical attention. Avoid ointments, antiseptic liquids or powders (which may react with the chemical) until after the injury has been assessed by a medical professional. Later, washing with lungwort decoctions is good for damaged skin.

- *Splash into eye(s)* – a prolonged (10–15 minutes) rinse with clean water with eyelids held open, is required. Cover the affected eye(s) with clean gauze and seek medical attention.

- *Burns and skin contact* – follow the procedures for *spill/ splash/skin contact* and *splash into eye(s)* entries above. Poultices of ivy leaves have traditionally helped skin eruptions and sores, while the topically applied juice of certain grasses of the *Miscanthus* species – particularly *Miscanthus sinensis* – dissipates extravasated (leaked into the tissues) blood if required.

- *Inhalation* – move the casualty into the fresh air. If the chemicals are safe to dilute (check the label on the container), immediately rinse the mouth and nose with clean water. Call for an ambulance as inhalation can impact on the respiratory tract and chemicals can enter the bloodstream via the lungs, and delayed respiratory problems or triggered cardiac arrest can occur.

- *Swallowed* – call the emergency services. Rinse the mouth and then gargle the throat with clean water – swallowed chemicals may harm the digestive tract but they can trigger more widespread damage if they enter the bloodstream. If a corrosive substance (check the label on the container) is swallowed, drinking water or milk may dilute it, but check with poisons control before doing this. While waiting for the ambulance, find out the name of the chemical, how much was swallowed, and whether it was diluted or not. This will be helpful to the paramedics and doctors.

KNOCKS AND BUMPS

The garden is as good a place as any to pick up a few knocks
and bumps; as gardeners, we spend more time in it than on
a big soft couch (safe and out of harm's way). These knocks
may be simple mishaps, such as walking into a low branch, for
example, but often they are task- or tool-related. Some, such
as stepping on a rake and piercing your foot – are covered
in detail in the 'Common garden accidents' section (see page
159ff), but, for now, here are some general bumps along the
road to a perfect garden.

BANGED ELBOW, KNEE OR SHIN

The first action should be to rub the affected area – this
disrupts sensation receptors and is very effective. Then walk it
off – get on with what you were doing as this gives the brain
something else to focus on, engages other neurotransmitters
and steps off the pain agenda more quickly. The aescin found
in a tincture or paste of horse chestnut can ease pain, swelling
and bruising – great also for tired legs and muscle cramps.
Wintergreen is pain-relieving when absorbed through the
skin.

KNOCKED OUT

If it is safe to do so, place the casualty in the recovery position
and dial the emergency services. If it is you that has been
knocked out, get to hospital for a check-up when you regain
consciousness.

Creeping Jenny and Ground Ivy Bruise Buster

Both creeping jenny and ground ivy are considered weeds in a garden context, but they are nonetheless helpful, as creeping jenny is astringent and calming, while ground ivy is soothing, astringent and has a toning action. Both are packed with the right sorts of tannins to remedy any bruise. Tannins shrink swollen tissue and narrow blood vessels, thus helping to diminish bruises.

METHOD

Locate these plants in your garden and simply squeeze some sap from their leaves and stems and dab the area around the bruise with the juice. If using around the eye area, do not let the sap make contact with the eye itself. Repeat a few times daily to shrink the bruise in no time.

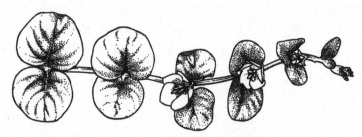

Creeping Jenny

KNOCKED-OUT TOOTH

A chipped tooth may mean a visit to the dentist but a knocked-out tooth requires a trip to the dental hospital or your local emergency room for re-implantation. Pop the tooth in a glass of milk (this preserves it and cleanses it of fungal or bacterial debris) and stem any bleeding in the mouth (a refrigerated moist cloth strip works a treat) before taking the casualty plus the glass of milk with the tooth to the dentist/doctor. But don't get thirsty and drink the milk on the way!

TRIPS AND FALLS

Be it a trip, slip or even a fall from a ladder, the protocol is the same: don't move, take a breath, be calm and get your bearings – are you hurt, or just embarrassed and winded? If the latter, get up, but not too quickly, as some injuries are only revealed when you try to stand. If you are badly hurt, or any of your limbs feel numb, call for help and the emergency services; do not move and stay calm until help arrives.

If you are hurt but feel it is not too serious, then roll onto your hands and knees, assess the situation from this position and decide whether you are able to stand. On standing you may discover that you have hurt your back, buttocks, knee or other point of contact with the ground – address these injuries from home unless blood flow or breaks require a first response on site. If on standing there is no further pain, take a rest anyway. If you banged your head, seek medical assistance and have a check-up. Falls may result in breaks (see page 151) or sprains (page 87), and if bleeding after a fall, see page 112.

They say that if you forget to hit the ground when you fall, you fly. Well, some accidents just knock the wind out of you and some cause embarrassment. One way of flying again is to smell the roses – literally, go over and take a sniff. The aromas in your garden can flood out pain receptors and reboot the positive brain. If you are in need of a reaffirming boost, head for your favourite fragrance. If treating a casualty, then the inhalation of the fragrance of lavender or mint can energise, while the fragrance of lilac can tranquillise. Rose petal tea is a pleasant pick-me-up (forgive the pun) after a fall, provided there are no injuries which require hospital treatment. In the latter case, it must be 'nil by mouth' until the casualty has been assessed by medical personnel.

BLACK EYE

Stepped on a rake while shooing the pigeons off your cabbages? Had an apple conk you in the face while harvesting the last of the higher fruits? Whatever the mishap, the first response is the same – cool the bruise as soon as possible after the injury.

A black eye is simply impact swelling and bruising to tissue under the skin surrounding the eye. The surface skin becomes 'black' (generally bluish or purple) because tiny skin blood vessels have burst and leaked a little blood out into the surrounding soft tissue. It is not a serious injury and heals naturally. If it was a particularly nasty impact that caused the black eye then always take a precautionary look for any signs of bleeding or damage to the white of the eye and note any pupil abnormalities – if either is found or there are vision difficulties seek further medical assistance. A black eye usually takes about fourteen days to heal completely, but the process can be speeded up with some applied tannin via the garden or the kitchen – a moistened tea bag will do the job.

FIRST RESPONSE

Whether you use ice cubes or a bag of frozen peas (they don't have to be black-eyed peas!) the trick is to wrap the cooling object in a tea towel (direct frozen contact can undo the healing aim). Using gentle pressure, hold the cold pack in place, but do not press on the eye itself. The chill factor is anti-inflammatory and will also numb pain. Keep the pack on for 10–15 minutes at a time and repeat the process several times throughout the day for 24 to 48 hours.

GARDEN AID

Quite a few plants have the potential to shrink a bruise: arnica, creeping jenny, ground ivy and so on – simply made using the same method as any tincture recipe in this book and dabbed onto a cotton pad compress, or for expediency mash up some leaves of any of these plants to yield a sap gel and apply topically. This treatment is for a skin bruise, so avoid contact with the eye surface. Drinking a cup of tea while sitting on your favourite garden seat with the tannin-rich tea bag on your eye works a treat too. Rosewater or witch hazel compresses are soothing.

141

Black Tea Black Eye Compress

If your garden is 100 per cent weed free, this is a good alternative. The average tea bag is packed with tannins that reduce inflammation and remedy damaged blood vessels, and their bioflavonoid content also reduces inflammation and helps to inhibit discolouration.

METHOD

Make a cup of tea without milk or sugar. Lift out the tea bag but do not squeeze off the excess fluid, just place it on a saucer to cool (you may go on to make your tea as normal, with a little extra sweetness for the shock factor). When cooled enough to be safely left on the skin, apply the cool, wet tea bag over the eye as you would with a cucumber slice and relax while it works its magic. It may take a few cuppas over a few days but it will speed healing more quickly than doing nothing.

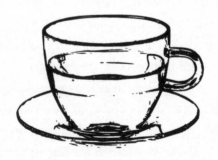

OTHER BRUISES/BUMPS

A bruise is the result of trapped blood that appears as the black-and-blue mark – the gardener's tattoo you could call it – and we perhaps would not know ourselves without one. I have perfected their cultivation alongside my endeavours to cultivate perfection in the garden. Bruises naturally heal in a few days to a fortnight but you can help the process along.

FIRST RESPONSE ✛

Apply a cold pack several times a day for a day or two after the initial injury. After that, heat packs can help to dissipate the trapped blood and speed up the natural healing process.

GARDEN AID

Use plants which discourage inflammation or the development of a haematoma (the blood leak and blueing part), or encourage faster fading of the bruise. Oil infuse some mullein flowers or crush in a mortar and pestle with some olive oil to yield a reviving oil. Try a comfrey compress after ice has been used, or a parsley compress at any time. A cotton pad soaked in chilled witch hazel extract and used as a compress helps to resolve bruises. Arnica is a brilliant bruise resolver, as is St John's wort – a paste, compress or tincture of either will work wonders. Golden loosestrife was long employed as a haemostatic and astringent, and the topically applied juice of *Miscanthus sinensis* is beneficial in dissolving blood coagulations and dissipating extravasated (leaked into the tissues) blood.

KITCHEN AID

A spritz or dab of vinegar will increase blood flow near the skin's surface and so contribute to dissipating the trapped blood.

Bruise Cure Tincture of Arnica, Calendula and St John's Wort

Tinctures are alcohol-based remedies that can be taken orally or used as a rub – this recipe is intended as a rub. This particular combination diminishes swelling and promotes fast resolution and fading of the bruise. Also good for aches, pains, sprains, cuts, scrapes and skin complaints.

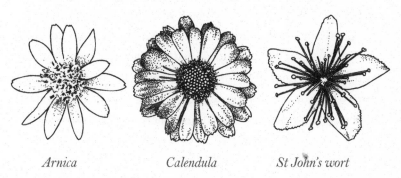

Arnica   *Calendula*   *St John's wort*

INGREDIENTS

½ cup arnica flowers and leaves

½ cup St John's wort flowers and leaves

¼ cup calendula flowers

1 cup vodka

METHOD

Using an airtight jar or container, soak all the ingredient plant parts (torn to release healing principles) in the alcohol on a sunny window sill for two weeks. Then strain the liquid and store in an airtight dark glass bottle in a dry cupboard.

This will store for several months. Shake well before use. This is definitely a 'here's one I made earlier' remedy – your bruise would be gone before the tincture is ready if you had to start from scratch, but it is worth making for all those bruises to come.

You can cheat a week off the steeping time of tinctures by making as an oil – using almost all the same ingredients, but replace the alcohol with oil. Simply warm any kitchen vegetable oil gently in a bain-marie and soak the herbs in it, decant into a clear bottle or jar and allow to sit on a sunny window sill for a week. The ratio of herb to oil is optional, but I like 1:2. A same-day hot oil infusion will have some impact once cooled and settled overnight, but tradition dictates a decent soak in the sun for the volatile oils to really penetrate the carrier oil.

In the meantime, try an even quicker fix:

Quick-fix Basic Bruise Mix

Take a tablespoon of each herb in the ingredients list for the tincture, chop them well, then add to 3 tablespoons of carrier oil (olive or other vitamin E-rich base) and a teaspoon of vinegar (any sort), then crush in a mortar and pestle into as creamy a paste as you can get. Stir your finger in the mix to get a coating of the medicated oil and apply to the bruise. Re-apply as needed. The mixture keeps for a week in the fridge (bonus chill factor). Simply re-stir well for subsequent applications.

Head bumps and other minor head injuries

Be it a bump, a bruise-producing knock or a scrape from a low-hanging branch, a gardener's head can often be above the parapet. The scalp is filled with blood vessels and may bleed excessively, even with the smallest wound or shallowest cut, but at the same time not be life-threatening. A small knock can trigger a big headache, though.

A head bump is not a minor injury if the casualty experiences any of the following: loss of consciousness, seizure, weakness on one side of the body, heart palpitations, unequal-sized pupils, vomiting, drowsiness, dizziness, confusion or a worsening headache.

First response

- If there is a cut, stem the blood loss then clean the wound and protect with a bandage or adhesive plaster.
- If there is a bruise, cold treat and see page 145–6 for remedies.
- If it is a bump or a knock that causes a slight headache, rest and take an over-the-counter or herbal painkiller.
- If the bump was with such force that it results in nausea and/or dizziness, then see a GP.
- If it was with such force that it knocked the casualty unconscious or left him or her seriously dazed or disorientated, then medical intervention is advised.

Never move unconscious casualties unless remaining in place puts them in serious jeopardy (from fire, flood, etc.).

147

GARDEN AID

The bark, leaves and twigs of the Salix (willow) species contain salicylic acid, which reduces fever, pain and swelling, and can be used to make a medicinal tea, as can meadowsweet (once known as *Spiraea ulmaria* – providing the *spir* part of the word aspirin), which makes a sweeter herbal tea – both can be applied topically in compress form too. Topically applied yarrow juice or its crushed leaves can staunch blood flow, and a thyme tea will clean wounds.

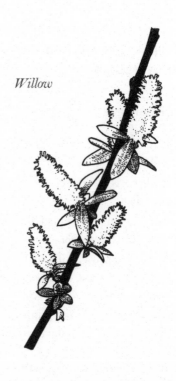

Willow

STUBBED TOE AND NAIL BED BRUISES

Open-toed sandals are all well and good for enjoying the garden, but not for working in it – and it is all too easy to stub a toe in the winter even in better protective footwear. A trip or an object falling on the foot can bruise, cut, break or dislocate a toe.

STUBBED TOE

Any mishap where you strike a toe against a hard object is painful for a few moments and then passes without much attention being paid, but occasionally the force of impact is strong enough to cause the toe to swell and even bruise the flesh – or worse, instigate a nail bed bruise.

FIRST RESPONSE

Apply ice, elevate the injured foot – and rest for a while.

GARDEN AID

Any of the bruise or anti-inflammatory remedies will help (see pages 145–6). Topically applied Sedum juice is astringent, as are boiled privet leaves in poultice form. Purple loosestrife is rich in tannin and can make a rinse or compress, and a poultice of acanthus leaves or comfrey can strengthen the injured toe and speed recovery.

Nail bed bruise (subungual haematoma)

A direct blow or injury to the toenail can cause blood loss from capillaries under the nail bed – the pressure generated by the accumulation of blood and swelling from the impact can cause intense pain.

First response

Cold therapy and a GP visit in case draining is required – if the nail was removed by the injury or subsequently falls off, then an antiseptic wash and a dry, sterile bandage (or adhesive plaster) is called for.

Garden aid

Bird's foot trefoil may be used as an anti-inflammatory compress – if mixed in a mortar and pestle with equal parts arnica and witch hazel it can make a fine dissipater of clots or bruises, as well as reducing swelling. Golden loosestrife and purple loosestrife are strongly astringent and suitable for rinses, poultices or even made into salves.

BROKEN BONES/FRACTURES

It is not easy to break a bone while gardening unless you have a fall or something falls on you. The treatment response depends on which bone has been damaged, but three general guidelines are universal:

1. Immobilise the limb or body part with the break.
2. Get the casualty to a hospital for a proper diagnosis (and to ascertain whether there are any complications – a broken rib could puncture a lung, for example).
3. Nil by mouth in case there is need for a general anaesthetic to repair the fracture or deal with secondary injury. A 'fracture' is the medical definition of bone damage, from a hairline crack to a complete break.

FIRST RESPONSE

Immobilise the injured limb with a sling or splint and get the casualty to hospital for an X-ray and further treatment. For how to make a sling or splint, see pages 273–4.

GARDEN AID FOR ANY BREAKS

Continue to enjoy your garden while recovering from a break. Relax in the sun and try to have 15 minutes of sunshine on unprotected skin daily to boost your vitamin D levels, which will help with calcium absorption from your diet and the use of the calcium for bone healing. A dose of daylight also resets circadian rhythms in the brain, leading to more restful sleep and less night-time agitation of a broken limb, or twisting and turning over onto damaged bone.

COMMON BREAKS: BROKEN ANKLE

Twisting the ankle or tripping can easily lead to a broken ankle (generally the fibular bone), which can take four to eight weeks to heal properly. The severity of the pain is variable, but often emotional shock – leading to dizziness and nausea – can accompany a break that impairs mobility.

FIRST RESPONSE ✚

Immobilise the ankle with a splint and keep weight off it. Get the casualty to hospital for an X-ray and treatment. Ice packs or a bag of frozen vegetables may be useful to reduce swelling while waiting for an ambulance or en route to hospital.

COMMON BREAKS: BROKEN ARM

A fall or other collision-type force can break any of the bones in the arm. Arm bones can take anywhere from six to eight weeks to heal fully. Pain is generally moderate to severe on movement.

FIRST RESPONSE ✚

Immobilise the arm by employing a sling (a towel or t-shirt improvised under the arm and then around the neck will suffice). Ice packs can help to reduce swelling and numb pain. Get the casualty to hospital for an X-ray and further treatment.

COMMON BREAKS: BROKEN COLLARBONE/ CLAVICLE

This can be extremely painful with the slightest movement, especially as the collarbone no longer provides support so the shoulder is often pulled downwards and forward under the weight of the arm. It will take six to eight weeks to heal the bone and possibly a further four-week recovery period.

FIRST RESPONSE

Use a sling and a belt to strap and immobilise the injured part. Adding an ice pack is optional, to reduce swelling and help to numb the pain. Get the casualty to hospital for an X-ray and further treatment.

COMMON BREAKS: BROKEN FOOT/TOE

It is amazing to think that nearly a quarter of all the bones in the human body are located in the feet. Forefoot bones (metatarsals) and toe bones (phalanges) can potentially fracture through the dropping of a heavy plant pot or other weighty object on the foot or striking the toe against a hard surface. Toe fractures can take four to six weeks to heal completely, but some may require professional reduction (realignment) first. Metatarsals can take longer and may need outpatient care.

153

FIRST RESPONSE ✚

If a toe is hurt, place some cotton wool or gauze between the injured toe and the one next to it and tape them together to use the unbroken toe as a splint. Ice will reduce pain and swelling. If the whole foot is hurt, splint and ice. With either injury, get the casualty to hospital for an X-ray.

FOR THE NEXT FOUR TYPES OF INJURY, AMATEUR INTERVENTION IS NOT ADVISED.

BROKEN HAND/FINGER

Of all breaks, this is the most serious, as use of the hands is vital in the garden, so any negligence in seeking medical intervention to realign breaks correctly can result in loss of dexterity and later pain or arthritic-type symptoms. The hand contains twenty-seven bones in total. The palm hosts five bones called the metacarpals; and the fingers comprise fourteen phalanges. The hand bones can heal fast enough but consult a GP or physiotherapist about exercises to speed recovery.

BROKEN LEG

Be it a tibia/fibula or femur fracture, this will require an X-ray, medical realignment and a cast, and perhaps even surgery. Splint and ice, and call an ambulance to take the casualty to hospital.

BROKEN NOSE

A fall or stepping on a rake can break a nose and the break might not be noticed – just some swelling and pain which are easily remedied with ice and painkillers. But if the nose is misshapen or crooked you can do more damage than good and leave yourself looking like a boxer who never won a bout. Let the professional attend to it. Ice it and get to the hospital.

BROKEN WRIST

There are eight bones called carpals in the wrist. The most common gardening fracture of the wrist is a distal radius fracture. Wrist fractures can take six to eight weeks to heal completely. Casts are often employed, and occasionally plates. An X-ray will be required to ascertain the full implication of the injury, so the best an amateur can do is to splint, sling and ice the injured limb en route to hospital.

Remedies Beneficial to Broken Bones

A nice cup of tea

Green tea with jasmine can prime the body for healing; gingko boosts circulation and will help to flush toxins and haematomas away from the injury site. Horsetail tea is high in silica, which helps to restore bone tissue and improves calcium absorption. Alfalfa, burdock, chickweed, dandelion leaf, nettle and red raspberry tea are all mineral rich and help with bone setting and regeneration.

Cloth soaks

Positioned on/near the injury site, use a cloth wrap soaked in a decoction of one or more of any of the following: willow leaves, oak bark, marshmallow root, mullein herb, horsetail, wormwood, lobelia, skullcap and comfrey root. All of these are beneficial to bone and tissue regeneration. The cloth wrap can be chilled in the fridge to cool inflammation and to ease the itch factor.

Horsetail

Bathtub soaks (after cast removal)

Have a warm bath with added Epsom salts and some herb and floral additions that release healing agents beneficial to bone repair and tissue regeneration, as well as soothing itchiness and other skin irritations. Try any of the following: calendula, camomile, comfrey, horsetail, juniper berries, mullein, willow and rosemary.

Functional food

Vitamin K, found in vegetables and in particular in leafy greens, will speed recovery and strengthen bones, and the power of oats to regenerate and to mildly sedate makes porridge, flapjacks, oat muffins and even oat tincture from your local pharmacy or homemade, taken in your favourite beverage, a great support in dealing with fractures. Their gentle, calming effects ease the agitation and tedium of the long recovery period.

Comfrey

This herb, also known as 'knit bone' and 'boneset', has a long history of use in the treatment of broken bones. It was once prescribed to be taken internally because of its potent constituents of calcium, vitamins B12, A and C, potassium, iron, phosphorus and selenium, but it has come to light in recent decades that it also contains pyrrolizidine alkaloids that unfortunately damage the liver. If comfrey tea or steamed comfrey and cabbage is currently off the menu, in poultice form it is not: comfrey leaves and roots contain allantoin, a substance that promotes cellular growth and reduces inflammation, not to mention the absorption of all of its other healthy compounds. Comfrey root mash was once used to make casts in the days before the use of plaster of Paris.

157

Pretty picks

Columbine root paste was once a popular remedy for relieving rheumatic aches and joint pains and may have an application to post-break recovery, while the dried leaves of mock orange can be mixed with witch hazel or a carrier oil to treat swollen joints, joint fractures and cast sores.

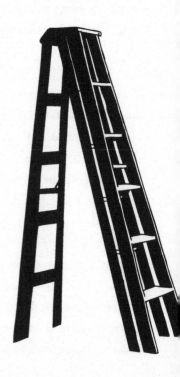

COMMON GARDEN ACCIDENTS

Accidents happen easily in the garden, including some that you pray will never happen. Most can be limited (in frequency and in potential damage) by the use of personal protective clothing – you may lose a toe if you are wearing scandals, but rarely would you do so in tough boots, and it's harder to cut a finger through a glove or poke an eye when wearing goggles. That said, I have been cut, stung, pricked, scalded and pinched more times when having lunch or drinks in other people's gardens (what does that say about me?) than when working in my own – and a 'dress casual' invitation does not include wearing protective clothing.

When it comes to most common garden accidents, the top ten offenders are the following gardening implements:

1. Lawnmowers (including back strain and finger nicks, as well as more serious injuries).
2. Flowerpots and planters (including falling over, dropping and lifting accidents).
3. Shears, secateurs and other manual pruners – plus knives and scissors.
4. Spades and forks.
5. Electric hedge trimmers.
6. Hoses and sprinklers.
7. Garden canes and sticks.
8. Rakes and hoes (stepping on and back strain).
9. Step ladders and ladders.
10. Items associated with alfresco cooking.

DISLOCATION

Dislocation is a serious injury and requires prompt, professional medical intervention to realign the bones that were forced from their normal positions when the injury occurred – usually a fall in gardening terms. Shoulders and elbows are most vulnerable, but thumb dislocations are also possible (see 'fingers and thumbs', page 163). Pain can be quite severe. A visit to the hospital is required.

FIRST RESPONSE

Immobilise the injured joint with a splint – do not try to move the joint back into place as incorrect manipulation can damage the surrounding muscles and ligaments and the injury may be complicated by proximity to nerves or blood vessels. Use cold therapy/an icepack to numb pain, reduce swelling and delay fluid build-up.

GARDEN AID

The roots of tree peony are antimicrobial, anti-inflammatory, analgesic, sedative and anticonvulsant, and in poultices and decoctions may be beneficial to arthritic joint swelling and other joint injuries. Garden peonies can also play a role through their painkilling action – delivered via soups, tisanes or decoctions (see pages 132–3 for other peony preparations). An astringent and emollient paste produced from the roots and/or leaves of acanthus was used in the past to aid the repositioning and healing of dislocated joints, pulled muscles and ligament strains.

SLICE THROUGH TOE/TOE AMPUTATION

The classic toe amputation scenario is to slice it off with a sharp spade – but scything, mowing or strimming while wearing open-toed sandals are not unknown mishaps. Toe tips are packed with nerve endings and blood vessels, so pain and blood loss is inevitable. Replantation may be possible, but the first call is to stop blood loss and get medical assistance.

FIRST RESPONSE FOR A PARTIALLY SEVERED TOE

Stop bleeding, protect the wound and get medical assistance. Cover the toe-tip wound with a slightly moist sterile dressing and wrap the whole foot with a bandage to immobilise and protect the damaged part. Elevate the injury. Holding a cold pack to the damaged foot while waiting for the ambulance can help to reduce bleeding and swelling. If bleeding is profuse, apply pressure just back from the severed point to stem the flow – see page 254.

FIRST RESPONSE FOR A FULLY AMPUTATED TOE

Stop/stem the blood flow – apply pressure and bandage wrap the open wound as above. Call for help and an ambulance.

Top tip

To save the severed toe, rinse the toe clean, wrap it in cling film or moist gauze, place inside a ziplock-type plastic bag, put that bag inside a container packed with ice or frozen vegetables and take it to the emergency room or give to paramedics.

GARDEN AID

Here we are restricted to recovery support after the wound has been treated, by using herbal teas and compresses to promote peripheral blood flow. As an edible herbal option, both hawthorn and gingko are very effective, but also consider evening primrose oil and other agents rich in omega-3 fatty acids to add to your diet to inhibit post-surgery constriction of the small blood vessels and prevent rejection.

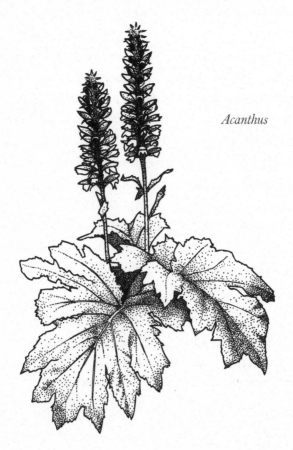

Acanthus

FINGERS AND THUMBS

Sometimes one can be all fingers and thumbs in the garden, and far from being green, they end up black and blue. Here are the four most common inconveniences that affect the digits.

JAMMED FINGER/CAUGHT FINGER

It doesn't have to be jammed in a shed door, but might be pinched between two sleepers or bricks during a construction project or caught while repositioning a plant pot or garden furniture. A jammed finger can be anything from slight pinch pressure to a crush injury requiring medical attention, but most frequently it happens as a not too serious impact injury that results in joint pain and immediate inflammation.

FIRST RESPONSE ✚

Cold therapy (for 10 minutes at a time) and elevation of the finger are advised, but if after a few chill sessions the pain is gaining intensity or the finger cannot be flexed, even slightly, then an X-ray should be sought to check for a fracture. Once the swelling subsides there are usually no more complications and most caught fingers heal in a day or two. Some jammed fingers (especially the car door type) can result in fracture or dislocation.

DIGIT DISLOCATIONS/DISLOCATED FINGER

A finger dislocation requires medical intervention to put the joint back into place – generally by reduction and splint but occasionally surgery is required.

First response ✚

Remove any rings and apply ice to reduce swelling. Elevate the finger above the heart and seek medical assistance. Home splinting can complicate the injury, so use a sling instead to support the injured limb.

Garden aid

The tincture and paste of the rhizome of blue flag iris treats rheumatism and joint pains, while the roots of tree peony are anti-inflammatory, analgesic, sedative and anticonvulsant and so are beneficial to arthritic joint swelling and other joint injuries.

Hammered thumb/struck thumb

There is a brachydactylic or stumpy thumb condition that is often referred to as 'hammer thumb', but here hammered thumb refers to a mishap where you hit your thumb with a hammer – resulting in pain, inflammation and a black nail bed bruise.

First response ✚

Ice and elevation – if black fingernail develops or the pressure/pain is too strong it may be necessary to consult a GP.

Black fingernail

Not the dirt or the evidence of gardening activity but a sub-ungual haematoma or nail bed bruise resulting from a direct blow or injury to the fingernail and blood loss from capillaries under the nail bed. The pressure generated by the accumulation of blood and the impact swelling can cause intense pain.

FIRST RESPONSE ✚

Cold therapy and a GP visit in case draining is required. If the nail was removed by the injury or subsequently falls off, then an antiseptic wash and a dry sterile bandage (or adhesive plaster) is called for.

GARDEN AID

Bird's foot trefoil is also known as 'Fingers and thumbs' and may be used as an anti-inflammatory compress in cases of skin inflammation.

Fingers and Thumbs Unguent

Gather ⅓ of a cup of bird's foot trefoil and make a paste in a mortar and pestle with equal parts of arnica and witch hazel to use as an ointment. It is a bruise-shrinking as well as swelling-reducing remedy for any of the above 'finger and thumb' injuries.

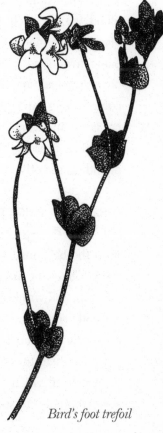

Bird's foot trefoil

Severed digits — finger and fingertip amputations, including thumbs

The classic finger amputation scenario takes place when clearing debris from a lawnmower or hedge-trimming equipment while the power is still on (and sadly those fingers affected are often so mangled or contaminated that reattachment is impossible), but mishaps with other garden implements can fully or partially sever a finger.

Because fingers and fingertips are rich with nerves and blood vessels such an accident can be quite a painful and bloody experience. When dealing with such a situation, don't panic, avoid shock and get help. In many cases, fingers can be reattached, most tip injuries grow over without much complication, and half-severed or hanging finger ends can be saved in many cases. That said, full recovery may take several months or permanent side-effects may be experienced, including sensitivity to cold or reduced dexterity.

First response for partially severed finger or thumb ⊕

Stop the bleeding, protect the wound and get medical assistance. Cover the fingertip wound with a slightly moist, sterile dressing and wrap the whole hand with a bandage to immobilise and protect the damaged digit. Elevate the injury. Holding a cold pack to the damaged hand while waiting for an ambulance can help to reduce bleeding and swelling. If bleeding is profuse you will need to apply pressure just back from the severed point – to stem the flow – see page 254.

FIRST RESPONSE FOR FULLY AMPUTATED FINGER OR THUMB ⊕

Stop/stem the blood flow – use pressure point technique (see page 254) if dressings plus pressure are not working. Call for help and an ambulance. Prepare the amputated finger/thumb part for potential reattachment – gently and briefly rinse the amputated part with water, wrap in a damp tea towel, moist gauze or cling film, then place in a re-sealable or watertight bag. Place that bag on ice (put it in a second bag, basin or container with ice and water or a pack of frozen vegetables) and take to the emergency room or give to paramedics.

> ### *Top tip*
>
> *Never put the amputated part directly in contact with the ice or frozen material as that could cause further damage.*

GARDEN AID

Recovery support is available from the garden: gingko and many other herbal teas can promote blood flow to reattached digits and prevent inflammation and rejection. Compresses of circulatory and antiseptic herbs can be used within days of surgery.

SEVERED LIMB

This type of accident is caused most commonly by a chainsaw or shredding device. The loss of an arm or leg – be it below or above a joint – is a serious and life-threatening trauma, both through the potential for serious blood loss and through shock.

Note: A tourniquet is a last-ditch option and should not be used unless a pressure dressing has failed to stop the bleeding and the casualty is in danger of bleeding to death before the ambulance service arrives. An improvised tourniquet can potentially damage blood vessels and nerves. If you are forced to use one, then use a belt or strap, not wire or a shoelace – once applied, do not loosen or release the tourniquet until medical assistance arrives.

FIRST RESPONSE

- Call the emergency services.

- Control bleeding – to staunch blood flow, cover the open wound with a moistened sterile dressing (a tea towel will suffice), apply direct and firm pressure over the bleeding site and elevate (if possible) the severed limb above the level of the heart.

- Use pressure points (see page 254) to further slow blood loss – over the brachial artery for the arm and femoral artery for the leg.

- Minimise movement of the injured limb.

- Watch out for shock symptoms (see page 214) and apply suitable treatment.

- Prepare to administer CPR if required.

- If possible, gather the amputated body part and place in a clean plastic bag that can be tied off to become watertight, or wrap in cling film. Place the bagged limb inside another bag containing ice/pack(s) of frozen vegetables – never put a severed limb directly onto ice as it can damage the tissues and complicate potential reattachment.

Splinters

Even without the carpentry projects that gardening sometimes entails, there are wooden artefacts that we encounter regularly – everything from tools to plant supports to boundary fences – but a splinter doesn't have to be made of wood: a microscopic shard of plastic, a sliver of glass or even a metal fragment can penetrate the skin, occasionally even through gloves or clothing. Tie-in wire and plant spines are my regulars.

The term 'splinter' generally denotes an embedded object, with the potential risk of secondary infection, so while the injury is initially painful through the piercing of skin or ripping of flesh, the main concern is removal of the splinter and antiseptic treatment.

First response

Rinse the damaged area under a tap or gently clean the area with mild soap and water, with a dash of antiseptic liquid, then, if the object is protruding, remove it slowly with sterile tweezers and afterwards re-apply antiseptic. Use an adhesive plaster to keep the puncture wound clean while it heals over. If the object is not protruding enough to get a grip on it, most small splinters will work their own way out over a few days, or you could try a hot poultice of bread, oats or a cabbage leaf, or make a drawing salve to encourage it out more quickly.

Sometimes with larger embedded splinters there is a need to use a sterile sewing needle to follow the path of the splinter and gently open enough skin to gain access with the sterile tweezers. Very large or deeply embedded splinters may need

170

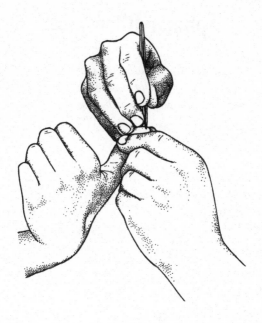

medical supervision or the skills of a local GP. If the wound site is bleeding heavily, bandage the wound and seek medical assistance.

Even with the tiniest splinter, after extraction keep an eye on the site for any signs of infection – prolonged redness, further swelling, increasing pain, or pus at the site.

GARDEN AID

Any of the antiseptic ointments, salves or rinses described in this book are good for splinter recovery, but the garden is beneficial in yielding ingredients for drawing salves or leaves to steam as a drawing compress – for example, dock, comfrey and cabbage.

171

Splinter-lifter Salve

This is a 'drawing' salve, which helps to ease embedded shards up to the surface of the skin. It is good for skin in general and specifically for use with sundry puncture wounds, bites, stings and abrasions.

INGREDIENTS

- ⅓ cup each of calendula flowers, chopped comfrey leaves and plantain, dock or chickweed leaves (optional depending on which plants you have around – all these plants are remedial to skin and beneficial for drawing purposes)
- 2 cups olive oil (to infuse the above ingredients)
- 2 tablespoons honey
- 2 tablespoons coconut oil
- 2 tablespoons shea butter
- 25g pure beeswax, grated (the quantity can be amended to suit the preferred final consistency)
- 10 drops tea tree *or* eucalyptus essential oil
- 10 drops lavender essential oil
- 1 teaspoon vodka *or* rubbing alcohol

METHOD

In a bain-marie or in a Mason/Kilner jar standing in hot water, heat infuse the herb ingredients in the olive oil (by simmering for 1 hour minimum), then strain the herbs from the oil.

While the strained oil is still warm, take ⅓ of a cup of it* and stir in all the remaining ingredients, adding more infused oil if necessary to get the consistency right – gloopy, not paste-like. Reheat gently if needed to mix the beeswax through it thoroughly.

Decant into a suitable container, or leave it in the cup, and allow it to sit and stiffen (this may take an hour or two). Put a thick coating over the splinter site to draw the object out (it may take several applications to work the splinter to the surface).

Some people prefer their salves to be of a petroleum jelly or vapour rub consistency, while others prefer to harden them to resemble the texture of an old tin of shoe polish – you can achieve either by adjusting the beeswax to oil ratio. If it hardens to a more solid form than you like, just melt it again and add a little more oil, and if it is too soft, then reheat and add extra wax. If it ultimately sets too hard, just warm to a better consistency before applying.

The salve stores well in a cool dry place in an airtight container, with a longevity of several months. Use as needed.

* Keep the surplus oil for use in other salves and home remedies. As with culinary oils, check for rancidity (a stale smell or separation or discolouration) every couple of months, but it should last for years.

173

STEPPING ON A NAIL — AND OTHER GARDEN PUNCTURE WOUNDS

The most common gardening 'puncture wound' is stepping on a nail or treading on a sharp object hidden in the soil. A puncture wound normally only penetrates to a minor depth of skin/tissue and as such does not usually cause profuse bleeding. But if it does, see page 112.

Puncture wounds such as a mishap with a nail gun or falling on a garden cane are major injuries with the potential for internal bleeding and organ or blood vessel implications – call for help and the emergency services.

The more common garden type of puncture wound is rarely an embedded or splinter type but a piercing wound. For example, when a nail is stepped on, the nail normally does not remain in the wound, but comes out when the foot lifts off it. The wound may bleed, but the main issue is the risk of infection as the soles and foam inners of shoes can harbour bacteria, not to mention any bacteria from the soil on the puncturing object. See 'tetanus' on pages 178–9.

FIRST RESPONSE ✚

The first task will be to stop any bleeding by applying gentle pressure with a clean dressing. Once there is no sustained bleeding, clean the wound site and apply an antiseptic. Cover the wound with an adhesive plaster or a bandage to keep it clean. Change the dressing regularly and check for signs of infection (redness, swelling, oozing).

With any garden wound I recommend you consider the

injured person's tetanus status, but with foot wounds in particular, where the intruding object might have scraped against a bone, a medical check is the next port of call.

GARDEN AID

After all tetanus status and bleeding issues are resolved, an antibiotic foot bath is just the ticket. Make a strong pot of tea from yarrow, lavender, goldenseal and tilia/linden leaf (if you don't have one or more of these ingredients to hand, substitute with thyme, eucalyptus or mint). Add the pot of tea to a lukewarm foot bath with a heaped tablespoon of Epsom salts or bicarbonate of soda. All the ingredients are antibiotic and wound cleansing. This will also serve as a hand soak or bath additive.

STEPPING ON A RAKE

I paint all my garden tool handles bright red to avoid such scenarios – by making them easy to spot where I put them down when I get forgetful or busy. Red leaps out against the green of the lawn and the foliage of plants. However, such an accident can happen to the best of us, more often than we would like to admit, so there is no shame in stepping on a rake, but you have every sympathy if it hurts more than your pride or sense of safety consciousness.

If the implement punctures the foot, see wounds and tetanus entries on pages 270 and 178 respectively.

If it hits you in the face, as in a TV cartoon, it's time to get the 'acme' ice cubes out – see treatment for a black eye on page 140.

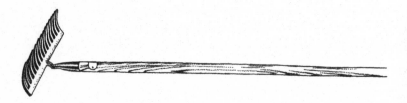

FIRST RESPONSE ✚

This is definitely one for a tirade of expletives, which is scientifically proven to lessen pain sensitivity, and personally I find it essential when I step on a rake or catch my thumb with a hammer, cursing myself as much as the implement. The next step is to address any bleeding or swelling – and usually after the injury wound care there comes an apology to the neighbours …

GARDEN AID

Make a sweet cup of tea, iced tea or a fruity beverage, sit in your favourite part of the garden and forget about it for 20 minutes. You will forgive the rake, forgive yourself and love the garden all over again ... until the next time.

Top tip

Don't make the iced tea a Long Island one (made with spirits) or let that fruity beverage become a cocktail. That leads only one way – to the next accident!

TETANUS/LOCKJAW

It's all about prevention with this one – glove up, take care with every cut and make sure you get your tetanus booster. The term tetanus describes both a bacterium (*Clostridium tetani*) and the name given to an acute infectious disease (contracted by contact with tetanus bacteria) which causes involuntary spasms of the muscles and jaw clamping – hence the disease's common name of lockjaw. It is not only rusty nail impalement or dog bites that can cause this lockjaw symptom – it can easily develop from wounds where flesh is torn (rather than neatly lacerated) or burnt. The recommendations regarding inoculations change regularly, but gardeners should have a booster if they haven't been inoculated against tetanus during the previous ten years.

Tetanus, as an anaerobic, spore-bearing, toxin-producing, gram-positive bacterium, has a worldwide distribution in soil, animal faeces (horse manure included) and even dust – all substances found in an average garden. Because the tetanus bacterium enters the human system via the types of cuts or wounds that gardeners regularly suffer, we are at higher risk of being infected than non-gardeners.

Tetanus symptoms manifest as painful muscles with accompanying stiffness (all over the body) and involuntary muscle tightening (often in the stomach or jaw). Trouble in swallowing, fever with sweating and seizures (jerking and/or staring) can arise too, alongside headache and high blood pressure with a fast heart rate. The incubation period from exposure to illness is usually three days to three weeks.

FIRST RESPONSE ⊕

Tetanus is a serious medical emergency requiring hospitalisation and medication that includes human tetanus immunoglobulin, strong antibiotics and anticonvulsive medicines to control muscle spasms, as well as treatments for secondary complications.

GARDEN AID

Build a healthy immune system with home-grown fruits and vegetables and cultivate a bed with the ingredients for body tonics and immunity-enhancing herbal teas – sage, camomile and mint – or whatever your favourites are. Passionflower tea (leaf infusion) has a reputation as an antispasmodic via its apigenin content. Linden tea is also antispasmodic and nervine – a nervine being a plant-based remedy that has a beneficial effect on the nervous system. Bistort root tea is used as a treatment in Chinese medicine. Japanese knotweed may prove useful too – try as tea or as a steamed vegetable.

Common garden eye injuries

Black eye
An astringent 'made and cooled' tea bag will do wonders for a black eye – see more on page 142.

Chemical splash in eye
Rinsing the eye with water for a minimum of 10 minutes is essential to dilute the chemical and stop it burning. See more on page 134.

Cuts around the eye
Tape a cotton pad or a layer of gauze over the eye, apply a cold pack and seek medical assistance. If there is bleeding, applying pressure is not advised, just hold the gauze padding gently but firmly in place but do not exert downward or inward pressure.

Embedded object
Be it a plant label, pencil, twig, splinter, rebounded nail, etc., do not try to pull it out. Cover the wounded eye and call an ambulance or take the casualty to hospital. Keep the good eye closed to minimise eye movement until help arrives.

Grit in the eye
Do not rub the affected eye, but pull the upper lid down over the lower lid and blink several times to dislodge any particles. If this does not work, try rinsing the eye with water for a few minutes and check with a mirror to see if you can manipulate

the grit to the inner corner. Once the grit is out use a cooled fennel seed and witch hazel extract cleansing eyewash (see page 183).

POKE IN THE EYE

If by a finger, and just a pressure injury, rest the eye with a cucumber slice or a cooled used tea bag as an eye pad. If the poke was with a stick, twig or sharp object, check for splinters/embedding or bleeding/cuts and follow the advice listed above.

ITCHY EYES

Use a fennel seed and witch hazel extract eyewash (see page 183).

SORE EYES

A distilled water prepared using the flowers of oxeye daisy is often used in eye complaints – especially with sore, tired, watery eyes, with styes and with conjunctivitis. Rosewater or witch hazel compresses are very soothing.

WATERY EYES

Try a cotton pad compress of camomile tea.

WEARY EYES

A compress of a slice of cucumber, raw potato or a strawberry will rejuvenate tired eyes. The closed-eye rest for the 20-minute duration of the compress will do no harm either. Rosewater or witch hazel compresses are also excellent.

Top tip

Eyesight is precious – always get eye injuries checked out – and do not judge the potential seriousness of an eye injury on the degree of pain experienced – e.g. alkali chemicals may not sting as much as acidic ones but can still destroy the tissues of the eye.

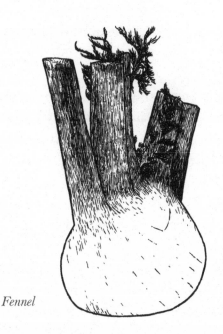

Fennel

Fennel Seed and Witch Hazel Good Vision Infusion

INGREDIENTS

Witch hazel extract (see page 188)
Fennel seeds
Salt
Water

METHOD

First make the witch hazel extract or buy a bottle from your local pharmacy or health store. Next, make an infusion of fennel seeds, using 2 tablespoons of seeds and one cup of boiling water. Crush or bruise the seeds with the back of a spoon and add to the freshly boiled water. Allow to steep for 20 minutes. While the seed tea is still hot, add a small pinch of salt to make the solution slightly saline and closer to the chemistry of tears. Strain the solids away and add two eggcups full (approx. 40ml) of witch hazel extract. Once the liquid reaches room temperature, rinse the eyes with the solution. The infusion will store for several days in the fridge.

Note: Cooled infusions of elderflower, eyebright, chickweed and camomile are all beneficial to eye health.

COMMON GARDEN MALADIES

We gardeners may succumb to wear and tear and occupational complaints now and then, or have to manage them on a long-term basis. Some problems may arise because of the way you work, but even with ergonomic practices some conditions are inevitable to those who are genetically prone – whether they are gardeners or not. But ergonomic practices can slow the onset of complaints, enable gardening to continue with such conditions or, for those not genetically liable, completely prevent symptoms from arising.

ERGONOMIC TIPS OF THE TRADE

- Wear gloves to protect your hands, not just from dirt and disease but also from blisters and calluses.

- Wear other personal protective gear appropriate to the task at hand.

- When using hand tools (trowels, shovels, rakes, hoes, etc.) try to keep your wrists as neutral as possible: over-gripping, over-extending or contorting angles may get the job done but injury will follow.

- Use the right tool for the job.

- Purchase tools with textured grips or padded handles for easier handling and, let's face it, better comfort.

- Sturdy tools are good but you don't need a big, heavy builder's barrow to move a few weeds to the heap or a set of pruners that bodybuilders would need a protein shake to operate.

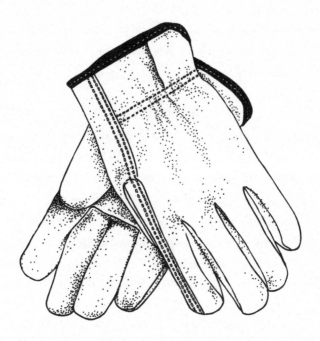

- Maintaining good posture while gardening is vital to maintaining a healthy back, but also to reduce stress on all ligaments, tendons, muscles and joints. Try to minimise bending, assuming awkward stances and stretching outwards or upwards.

- Kneeling is unavoidable, but always use knee pads or a cushioning device.

- Never risk straining your back when lifting; always bend the knees and use the strength of the thigh muscles.

- Don't over-exert yourself.

- Stay hydrated.

- Be weather conscious.

When it comes to general aches and pains, sprains and strains, pulls and pinches, see the 'Aches and pains' section starting on page 81.

BLISTERS

Blisters are small pockets of fluid that develop within the upper layers of the skin as a result of injury. While sunburn, thermal burns, freezing and chemical exposure can all result in blisters, for the most part gardeners suffer them from simple friction injuries – whether that is a too-tight shoe or a hard day for the hands with a pick or sledgehammer. Chores that can cause calluses can also cause blisters. Pinch injuries and jamming injuries can cause a blood-filled rather than fluid-filled blister, which is known as a blood blister (see page 190).

The sustained friction, by even something as mundane as raking without wearing gloves, causes a micro-tear between the upper layer of skin (epidermis) and the layers beneath; the breach becomes filled with plasma and swells to a bubble. Blisters resolve themselves naturally – as new skin grows underneath the blister, the body slowly reabsorbs the plasma and the bubble sac dries out and eventually falls off.

Top tip

Do not burst blisters – the unbroken skin over a blister seals the damage site and provides a natural barrier to contamination and infection. A dab of mouthwash (particularly Listerine) can encourage blisters to dry out and shrink more quickly.

First response ⊕

Rinse the blistered area under cool water to lessen swelling and clean the surface. Use a soft gauze or cotton pad under an adhesive plaster. 'Clean' and 'protect' are the watchwords.

If a blister bursts or becomes infected, use an antiseptic rinse or ointment and dress with some gauze and a breathable adhesive plaster.

Garden aid

The ever-useful sap of aloe vera or a squeeze of mint juice will benefit with its coolness and anti-inflammatory action. If you grow cucumbers, or have one in the fridge, then a chilled slice makes a brilliant cooling and regenerative compress for any blister. If the blister is large – say over the entire heel – then a cold compress of grated raw potato works a treat too. An infusion of the bark/leaves of the beech tree is antiseptic and astringent. The root of *Heuchera micrantha* (its common name of alum root is also a common name for geranium – so Latin here avoids confusion) is antiseptic and astringent. Horseradish root has a similar effect if you don't want to dig up a garden favourite. Witch hazel is a good tonic to apply to bruised and blistered skin.

Witch's Brew – Homemade Witch Hazel Extract

Traditionally, witch hazel extract was obtained by steaming the twigs of the shrub, but its leaves and flowers can also be used to extract the active principles of gallic acid, kaempferol, quercetin, catechins, proanthocyanins and eugenol as well as its tannin content – all of which are tonic, anti-inflammatory, antiseptic and astringent. This is a quick and easy recipe.

INGREDIENTS

Sprigs and twigs of the witch hazel bush (they are more potent when flowering and just after flowering)

Water

METHOD

Chop the sprigs and twigs up into rough sections and slice lengthways. Add to a pot with a tight-fitting lid, cover with double the amount of water to the herbage and bring to the boil. Cover, then simmer for a good six hours. You may need to add some fresh water occasionally if steam is escaping. Remove from the heat and allow to cool for one hour. Strain away the herbage and decant the liquid into clean bottles with corks or caps, or containers with tops.

The pure extract will keep for one week at room temperature or for several months if refrigerated. You can extend its shelf-life by adding some vodka to the mix, but for first aid purposes (and eyes) the pure tonic is sufficient and perhaps even superior.

Witch hazel extract is also beneficial as a skin toner, a soother of rashes and itching, pimple reduction, eye bag reduction, bruise shrinking and in treatments for varicose vein and haemorrhoid relief.

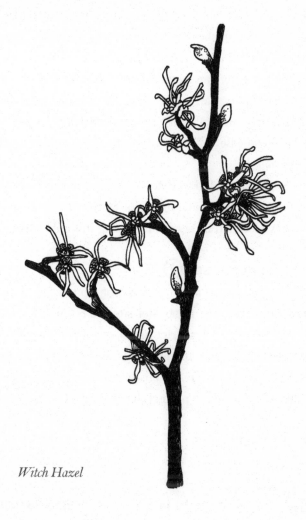

Witch Hazel

BLOOD BLISTER

A blood blister is what it says on the tin – a blister filled with some blood, usually from a rupture to a blood vessel below the injury but with no laceration to allow it to bleed freely. Like ordinary blisters, these come from friction or a pinch injury – tight shoes or a finger caught while laying slabs or moving wood, perhaps. There are a whole bunch of ways that a gardener can develop one – even the friction of a bit of arduous raking can trigger one. The trick is not to burst it. It will resolve naturally in a few days and pricking it, even with a sterile needle, will only make those few days a more painful experience.

Sometimes blood blisters accompany more serious complaints such as a burn injury or chemical splash and medical supervision will be needed following initial first aid for these.

FIRST RESPONSE

Rinse the affected area under a cool tap to clean it and reduce inflammation, then the blister site can be chilled to encourage blood vessels to constrict and so stop the internal bleeding and reduce further any inflammation. A chilled spoon will do the trick: place it on the blister for 10 minutes. Applying an adhesive plaster will protect the site and let it resolve naturally.

GARDEN AID

A squeeze of aloe or other succulent juice will cool and slow inflammation. You can, if the season is right, dig up a bulb of garlic and squeeze the juice of a single clove over the blood

190

blister. Garlic juice both disinfects and promotes subcutaneous healing. It needs to penetrate, though, so is best applied after chilling has lessened the size of the blister. Of course, the astringent tannins of witch hazel will dry out the blister and speed recovery, and a chilled yarrow tea will do wonders. The juices of both ajuga and cornflower are tannin rich and direct application or decoctions/compresses can shrink/treat blood blisters. Rhizome paste or tincture of cranesbill geranium is astringent. The juice of *Miscanthus sinensis* has a history as a refrigerant to cool fevers and as an anti-inflammatory, but it is also beneficial in dissolving blood coagulations and dissipating seeping blood, making it good for burns as well as blood blisters and bruises. Rosewater is a brilliant tonic for all forms of damaged skin (see page 192).

Rosewater

Rosewater is best made from freshly picked petals. I like to give the rose flower a gentle hose down on the bush to remove any insects and dirt particles and avoid wasting water. (I have generally tempered my holistic opinions up to now, but washing the flower on the plant is nicely ritualistic and you are watering the plant in thanks for its gift – it makes it more special, less of a pluck and run affair – in a way it sets the context for the spiritual and healing energy of the rosewater you will make.)

By the steeping method (infused water)

Harvest some roses (scented or not – the fragrance is not the vital part, only a bonus) and place their petals in a saucepan, adding just enough distilled/spring water to cover them. Bring to a simmer and keep your eye on the pan – we want steam but not a vigorous boil. Cover with a lid and allow it to simmer for a further 5 minutes then let it sit off the heat until the petals lose their colour and the water absorbs the roses' hue. You may notice some rose oil floating on the surface. Strain away the solids and decant the rosewater into a container. This will keep for two weeks if refrigerated.

By the distillation method (hydrosol)

This way is a bit more of a process, but worth it. First, construct a makeshift still, using a large saucepan, a slightly smaller lid, a cup, a small bowl and a tallish glass. Invert the cup in the centre of the saucepan; add the petals around it in the saucepan, plus enough water to cover them; the cup may still be visible depending on the quantity of roses used.

Balance the small bowl on top of the cup and place the tall glass in it as a support for the smaller lid (to be balanced on top of the glass), which will catch the steam and drip it down the sides of the glass into the gathering bowl. Bring the still to a simmer and keep it steaming, but not boiling hard, for long enough to gather a decent amount of steam-distilled essence. When the petals lose their colour you can stop distilling.

> ### *Top tip*
>
> *If the thought of balancing lids and bowls and cups and glasses gives you a feeling of panic, a simpler method I often employ is to use cling film as a lid, weighted with a stone in the centre – this dip funnels the drips into the gathering bowl.*

The rosewater keeps for two weeks in a fridge, or longer if converted into ice cubes – stick a fresh petal in each to identify.

The benefits of steam-instilled rosewater are well lauded but don't worry, as the steeping method yields the same healing properties. The advantage of steam distilling is that the residue left over in the pot at the end of the process is steeped method rosewater – so you get two for the price of one.

Calluses

They say hard work never killed anyone. I don't know about that, but hard work can harm: new projects, seasonal dig-overs, weeding blitzes and tool-heavy tasks can all generate callused hands.

A callus is just the thickening or hardening of the skin at points of friction or pressure. Calluses can appear on the palm of the hand and edge of the thumb, but most often with gardening, they develop at the base of the fingers – at the grip point for garden implements. Calluses are a natural defence mechanism against repeated friction and if they are not impairing dexterity or causing pain then removal or treatment is often seen as merely cosmetic – that said, though, there is no shame in having supple hands.

Corns and foot calluses

Some work boots are just not cut out for maintaining soft and supple feet – treat corns and calluses on feet as recommended below.

First response ⊕

Soften the skin with a soapy soak and exfoliate hard patches with a pumice stone. Never pare or cut away calluses.

Garden aid

A soothing salve of calendula and chickweed will soften calluses, as will a variety of skin-friendly lotions and creams manufactured from botanicals with emollient properties. Calluses can be softened with salicylic acid (willow, meadowsweet, etc.) and the top hard layer of dead skin pumiced or otherwise exfoliated away.

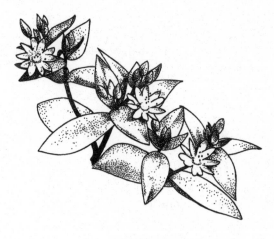

Chickweed

Calendula and Chickweed Salve

This combination packs a punch in treating a whole array of skin conditions including bruises, minor burns, cuts, scrapes and grazes, dry skin, chapped lips, sunburn and varicose veins.

INGREDIENTS

1½ cups olive oil or alternative carrier oil

1 cup fresh or dried calendula flowers

1 cup fresh leafy parts of chickweed

¼ cup shavings of pure beeswax (approx. 10–25g depending on the firmness of consistency preferred – the more wax, the harder the set)

Water to boil

YOU WILL ALSO NEED

A saucepan

Two glass Mason/Kilner jars or 2 Pyrex bowls

A wooden spoon or chopstick

Strainer/cheesecloth

A container to store the salve

METHOD

Wash and kitchen-towel dry your harvested herbs, then tear, crush or chop them to help release their active principles.

Place the herbs into a glass jar or Pyrex bowl and cover completely with the carrier oil. Attach the lid or seal the opening with cling film or kitchen parchment.

Bring a pan of water to the boil, then turn off the heat and stand the herb and oil-filled jar/bowl in the hot water and let it sit for 30 minutes to begin infusing.

After this, return the pan plus the jar/bowl to the heat and simmer for a further two hours, adding water to the pan as evaporation occurs. Then turn off the heat and allow the jar/bowl to sit in the hot water and continue to infuse for a further 30 minutes.

Strain off the herbs and decant the oil into the second jar/bowl. Chip, shave or grate the beeswax into the warm infused oil and stir until it dissolves, adding gentle heat via a bain-marie if needed.

Decant the mixture into your storage container and leave it to cool and solidify before lidding and storing for use.

The average shelf life of a homemade salve is approximately a year from the date you made it, as long as your base oil was fresh to begin with and thereafter it is stored in a cool location where it can remain semi-solid without continually re-melting and re-solidifying, thus spoiling.

Gardener's elbow/lateral epicondylitis

Lateral epicondylitis is commonly known as tennis elbow but this inflammatory condition affects gardeners too. A repetitive strain meets an occupational injury – triggered by twisting or gripping motions where the forearm muscles are contracted against resistance – such as using a screwdriver, pruning hedges or pulling weeds.

The lateral epicondyle is the bony prominence felt on the outside of the elbow – the condition occurs at the point where the tendon of the extensor muscles of the forearm meets it – from there, pain radiates to the forearm and often into the wrist. Grip strength can be affected and the simplest gardening chores become off limits. Early warning signs include morning stiffness in the elbow, slight swelling, tenderness, difficulty in fully extending the forearm and weakness in the wrist.

First response ⊕

PRICE (protect, rest, ice, compression and elevation) and more rest – supplemented with over-the-counter pain relief (aspirin or ibuprofen). Some sufferers benefit from an orthotic – be that a brace, band, splint or strap to stabilise the forearm and prevent a return to use until the elbow is sufficiently rested. If symptoms haven't resolved adequately in a couple of weeks, then a visit to a GP and some corticosteroid injections may be suggested.

Garden aid

Traditionally, calendula, camomile, eyebright, fennel, feverfew, meadowsweet and St John's wort are all anti-inflammatory herbs that can make a pleasing tea blend remedy or be used in salves or compresses for relief. A steamed cabbage compress is a remedy that can be used as a warm (heat) pack after cold therapy has ended. Wintergreen is best thought of as a topical aspirin – it is packed with salicylates.

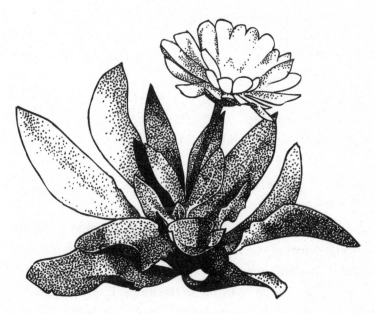

Calendula

Quick Blitz Gardener's Elbow Grease

A blender-friendly recipe for speedy results.

INGREDIENTS

- 4 tablespoons rubbing alcohol
- 4 tablespoons base carrier oil (olive, rapeseed, coconut, etc.)
- 2 tablespoons petroleum jelly (warmed to melt slightly – for a better mixing consistency) *or* supplement with any variety of aqueous solution, such as Silcock's base/E45 cream etc., or you can use castor oil
- 10 sorrel leaves, chopped
- 10 comfrey leaves, chopped
- 1 tablespoon ground fenugreek *or* a handful of sprouted fenugreek seeds
- 1 tablespoon turmeric
- 1 clove garlic
- ¼ cup strong, black camomile tea for use as a liquid to improve consistency

METHOD

Add the first eight ingredients with a few teaspoons of the strong camomile tea to a blender. Blitz to a paste consistency, slowly adding more tea until it reaches your preferred consistency. Jar up and store in the fridge. Use as required to reduce inflammation and treat the problem. Shake the mixture well before each use and use within a week.

Slather it on the affected joint and wrap with a bandage or gauze to keep it in place.

GARDENER'S KNEE/PREPATELLAR BURSITIS

There is a lot of kneeling and knee action going on daily as part of gardening – weeding, flexing to bend and lift, etc. – and occasionally praying for rain, or for the rain to stop. Gardeners can experience some pressure damage or swelling in the front of the knee which, with ongoing friction and activity, inevitably irritates the bursae (small lubricating sacs located just in front of the kneecap/patella), causing them to swell and become filled with fluid.

This condition is known medically as prepatellar bursitis. It is a form of repetitive strain injury and as an occupational injury is sometimes referred to as carpet layer's knee, housemaid's knee or, in our case, gardener's knee. Each knee has eleven bursae and any one of them is susceptible to bursitis from overuse.

The symptoms include inflammation of the kneecap and pain on activity, but not necessarily at night or at rest. The kneecap is generally tender to the touch and sometimes there is a warm sensation in the knee. Swelling can be dramatic on occasion. With rest and cold therapy, the problem generally resolves in a few days to a week. Prolonged inflamed periods or more frequent episodes will need a medical analysis and care regime.

FIRST RESPONSE ✚

PRICE (protect from further injury, rest, icepack, compression bandage and elevation) and anti-inflammatory medication (aspirin or ibuprofen). Prolonged cases may require a medical professional to aspirate the site, or, in severely debilitating cases, orthopaedic surgery. I have found that cold therapy three times daily for three to four days usually resolves the problem, but a follow-up with the same amount of heat therapy can delay repeat episodes.

GARDEN AID

Some willow bark tea will help to reduce the inflammation from both inside and out – have a cuppa to drink and one to make a compress. A tincture of Solomon's seal contains allantoin, a great skin aid and anti-inflammatory for connective tissues, which can be used internally or externally. A comfrey and willow leaf compress or mortar and pestle paste with a few drops of witch hazel or Solomon's seal tincture works a treat, or you could make a liniment (see recipe facing). Arnica tincture is effective in the relief of knee joint and muscle injuries, including gonarthrosis (disorder of the knee joint) and prepatellar bursitis.

Quick Blitz Gardener's Knee Liniment

A blender-friendly recipe for speedy results.

INGREDIENTS

½ cup rubbing alcohol

1 cup base carrier oil (olive, rapeseed, coconut, etc.)

¼ cup witch hazel extract

20 peppermint leaves

20 leaves Solomon's seal plus stem

10 comfrey leaves

2 sprigs rosemary (leaves only – discard the woody stem)

1 sprig lavender (leaves only – discard the woody stem)

1 tablespoon cayenne pepper

METHOD

Place all the ingredients in a blender and blitz to a liquid consistency. Jar up and store in the fridge. Use as required to cool and treat the problem knee. Shake well before use. Slather it on and wrap with a bandage to keep in place. Use within one week.

GARDENER'S WRIST/CARPAL TUNNEL SYNDROME

Gardener's wrist may be a simple ache from repetitive tasks on a given day or it may develop into a more concerted repetitive strain that affects the wrist nerves rather than the wrist muscles. As such it then becomes carpal tunnel syndrome (CTP), occurring when the tissues around the median nerve of the hand become inflamed and press on the nerve. This causes tingling at first, then pain and eventually weakness in the hand. Symptoms progress gradually over weeks, months or even years. If caught early, CTP symptoms are reversible, but if prolonged wear or overuse continues, then more permanent nerve damage may develop. Female gardeners have a significantly higher tendency towards carpal tunnel syndrome than their male counterparts.

FIRST RESPONSE ✚

On experiencing tingling, numbness or pain, consult your GP for an evaluation. Splinting will help to immobilise and reduce pain. Long-term treatment includes exercise to strengthen the mobility of the wrists, corticosteroid injections, and finally surgery.

GARDEN AID

Warmed comfrey and willow (*Salix spp.*) leaf compresses can follow cold therapy. Oil of St John's wort can be massaged into the wrists or a pad poultice of helichrysum oil is excellent. Infused oil of any or all of the above can be made into potent salves too.

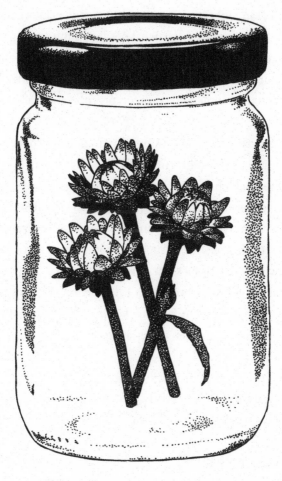

Helichrysum flowers inside a jam jar of oil

STRIMMER HANDS/HAND-ARM VIBRATION SYNDROME/VIBRATION WHITE FINGER

The use of any vibrating tool for prolonged periods in a given day can cause arm or hand weakness, numbness, tingling or tremor for a short period immediately after use. In the amenity horticulture trade these effects are known as strimmer hands – but a chainsaw, hedge trimmer or rotavator delivers the same effect.

The big risk is that prolonged vibrational exposure over many years can develop into HAVS – hand-arm vibration syndrome – which adversely affects the blood vessels, nerves, connective tissue, muscles and joints of the hand, wrist and arm. The repeated vibrations can cause the release of vasoconstricting chemicals such as serotonin and thromboxane into those nerves/tissues, etc. and over time damage them on a cellular level. One sure sign of HAVS is white fingertips, or fingers turning white or blue because of circulatory side-effects – hence the other common name of vibration white finger.

Some tools are more damaging than others – the most detrimental range is 5 to 20 Hz, which includes chainsaws and many other gardening tools.

FIRST RESPONSE ✛

Practice PR-W-CE (PRICE but without the ice – use warmth instead) and reduce (give up, if possible) exposure to vibrating tools. Specialist medical assistance is needed with more developed or repeated tremors and loss of dexterity – treatment may include calcium channel antagonists, physiotherapy and pain management.

GARDEN AID

Go low-tech – try no-dig gardening over mechanical tilling, use a scythe instead of a strimmer, and take up *o-karikomi* or other hand-shears topiary instead of regimented hedge lines. Let the lawn become a medicinal meadow full of clover, selfheal, bird's foot trefoil, camomile, etc.

If gardening is your occupation, invest in some anti-vibration gloves and hold vibrating tools as loosely as possible within health and safety requirements. Hold the tools in varying positions, and select low-vibration models. Take regular breaks of at least 15 minutes every hour – rebrand yourself as the low-tech gardening company or specialise in Zen gardens.

A pokeweed berry poultice is anti-rheumatic and helpful, and oil or liniment of wintergreen is packed with salicylate and acts rather like a topical aspirin. Both the pounded leaves of the well-known fragrant garden plant *Philadelphus* and applications of cottage garden staple columbine in root-paste form were once popular remedies to relieve joint pains.

Tai chi in the garden can benefit wrist and hand mobility.

KITCHEN AID

Bromelain, found in pineapple flesh and juice, inhibits kinins and other similar polypeptides – those natural bodily compounds that contribute to swelling – from working. Adding pineapple to a fruit salad, curry, pizza or other delicacy, adds an effective functional food for rheumatoid arthritis, osteomyelofibrosis and hand-arm vibration syndrome.

LIFE-THREATENING EVENTS

There are accidents and events that can potentially lead to loss of life – severed limbs, major bleeds, circulatory shock brought on by a severe burn or other injury and so on. Then there are those we may encounter without the apparent apparatus of catastrophe but which can nonetheless be catastrophic – stroke, heart attack, etc. So in this section are some of the dangerous events not previously covered that it is helpful to have some knowledge of, however they arise.

CHOKING/AIRWAY OBSTRUCTION – CONSCIOUS PERSON

If the capacity to speak or wheeze remains, that indicates an exchange of air, however diminished and however terrifying the sensation. A few strong coughs should dislodge the blockage – a piece of food, a swallowed insect, etc. If the casualty cannot speak, breathe or cough, then a full airway obstruction exists, necessitating use of the Heimlich manoeuvre. See 'coping with choking', page 263.

AIRWAY OBSTRUCTION – UNCONSCIOUS PERSON

Once a person is unconscious, muscles relax and if the casualty is left lying on his or her back, the tongue can easily fall backwards against the wall of the throat and impede air flow.

If safe to do so, putting the casualty in the recovery position and sweeping the mouth to reposition the tongue and check for other obstructions is traditional practice. See 'recovery positions', page 260.

ANAPHYLAXIS, ALSO KNOWN AS ANAPHYLACTIC SHOCK

This severe and often fatal allergic reaction occurs within minutes of contact with the trigger allergen (nuts, bee sting, etc.), and sometimes within seconds. In a garden context it arises most often from insect encounters.

FIRST RESPONSE

Call the emergency services. The effective antidote for anaphylaxis is an injection of adrenaline, which causes the blood vessels to constrict, raising blood pressure and reducing swelling, while triggering the airway to open, thus relieving any breathing difficulties. If a person has a previous history of anaphylaxis he or she will carry an auto-injector of adrenaline. Search their pockets and belongings for such an item. Injections are delivered into their thigh muscle (not the fatty part) and held in place for 10 seconds or until the adrenalin shot has fully dispersed.

Drowning/near drowning

A child can drown in as little as 5cm of water. The longer a child or adult is immersed in water, the more water is inhaled and swallowed, leading to loss of consciousness – so getting the casualty out of the water is crucial.

First response

Call for help and the emergency services. If possible, retrieve the drowning casualty or throw a buoyancy aid. Once the casualty is out of the water, clear and protect his or her airway. If he or she is breathing, protect from hypothermia until the ambulance arrives. If unconscious and not breathing, carry out CPR. If you are alone, the international recommendation is to perform CPR for one minute before calling for emergency help, then continue until an ambulance arrives. If the person is unconscious but still breathing, place in the recovery position, making sure that the head is lower than the body so that swallowed water can drain out.

Electrical shock/electrocution

The danger depends on the type of current and how high the voltage. But as even minor shocks can cause injury that ranges from numbness and tingling to heart arrhythmias, it is best to seek medical supervision after a shock. A major shock can be fatal.

First response ✛

Call the emergency services. Assess the scene with caution – is the casualty still in contact with the electrical source? Is the ground wet, or is the casualty on a conducting surface (metal ladder, etc.)? If any of these apply, if possible shut off the power supply at the mains. Never touch the person receiving the electric shock – electricity is a current and it will travel through you as well. If the current is no longer live, CPR or the recovery position may be required.

Head trauma/severe head injury

A serious bump or fall can occasion serious side-effects including loss of consciousness, seizure, weakness on one side of the body, heart palpitations, unequal sized pupils, vomiting, drowsiness, dizziness, confusion and debilitating headache. These may be signs of a fractured skull or a trauma to the brain and medical intervention is essential for proper diagnosis and treatment. Call the ambulance services. Do not remove any embedded object. Staunch bleeding without too much pressure – the brain can swell and fluid can build up under the concussive impact.

Heart attack

The majority of heart attacks occur in people over 45 years of age. Men are two to three times more likely to experience a heart attack than women. If you think that you or another person is having or has had a heart attack, call an ambulance. Even if symptoms subside, medical attention is essential.

FIRST RESPONSE

Have the casualty wait in the 'W-position' if possible (see page 261). If the casualty is not allergic to aspirin, slowly chewing a typical 300mg aspirin while waiting for the ambulance to arrive will help to thin the blood and thus restore a decent blood supply to the heart, easing pain and the clenched feeling. If the person becomes unconscious, clear the airway and, if necessary, start CPR (see page 256).

SEIZURE/FIT/CONVULSION

A strong seizure (grand mal) is the convulsive kind – limbs tremble and the body shakes, eyes may squeeze shut and facial contortion may be present. Such seizures can last for a couple of minutes, shutting off respiration, and the casualty may stop breathing for the duration of the fit, even turning blue. A weaker seizure or focal seizure (petit mal) is less dramatic to witness but nonetheless distressing to experience – the casualty may experience a tremor in one arm or body part and lose contact with perception/cognition/communication for a time – they may stare blankly for a few seconds and then come round.

FIRST RESPONSE

The aim is to protect the casualty rather than to 'control' the seizure. Move any dangerous or injurious objects out of the way, use a jacket to safeguard the casualty's head or act as a buffer between thrashing limbs and hard surfaces. Medical supervision is the next step for either seizure type – call the ambulance services.

SHOCK/CIRCULATORY SHOCK

Shock can be a feature of any garden injury. Circulatory shock is not the sensation of being shocked or taken aback by the injury – it is the failure of the cardiovascular system to maintain adequate blood circulation to the vital organs of the body (the heart, lungs and brain) during an injury event, and it can be fatal. The signs of shock can include anxiety and hyperactivity, but it generally manifests as stunned and distracted, with a fixed stare or vague look (pupils may be dilated), cool and clammy skin, often becoming pale or turning grey, an altered heart and pulse rate, breathing abnormality – shallow breaths or hyperventilation. The casualty may feel extremely weak and nauseated – they may even vomit. Shock indicates the body is shutting down.

FIRST RESPONSE ✚

Call the emergency services. Reassurance is key to bringing a person round; tell him or her firmly that everything will be all right. Laying the casualty down will improve circulation. Attend to any obvious injuries while waiting for the ambulance and keep the casualty warm with an extra coat or blanket – the aim is to avoid a drop in body temperature, but not to overheat.

Even if the casualty complains of thirst, *give nothing by mouth*. If the person stops breathing, start CPR and continue until the ambulance arrives.

STROKE

Stroke is a serious medical condition. Call the emergency services and reassure the casualty until the ambulance arrives. Even if symptoms dissipate while waiting for the ambulance, follow-up medical supervision is essential.

FIRST RESPONSE

Act fast; follow FAST – Face/Arms/Speech/Time – the quick guide to recognising signs and symptoms of a stroke, and seek medical attention. Drooping face, heavy or incapacitated arms or slurred speech mean it's time to call an ambulance. The earlier a casualty receives treatment, the better for long-term recovery.

WEATHER EMERGENCIES

As gardeners we are outside in all weathers and occasionally suffer the consequences of it – be it chilblained fingers or a sunburnt neck. The key to surviving all weathers is to have suitable clothing for all occasions but also to modify activities to match the weather – don't overwork in heat and don't dally in snow – all the common sense that we gardeners abandon when a tender plant needs to be wrapped, a rose needs pruning, a pond needs repairing or a squeaky wheel is needing attention.

Some underlying conditions are exacerbated by weather extremes, as pores open or veins constrict in response to heat or cold and the body suffers stress to compensate. Sometimes the weather can impact on how we act – forgetting to look after ourselves in the panic or pleasure of working in heatwave or monsoon conditions.

We can often work so hard and continuously to beat the weather that muscle fatigue or dehydration can set in, which can happen in any season, and in any climate. Both are best remedied with an isotonic drink – see page 242 for some recipes.

In the meantime, here are the more pernicious culprits to watch out for.

Hypothermia

Hypothermia officially occurs when a person's core body temperature drops below 35°C (95°F), but you know you are on the way if you have been exposed to extreme cold or a cold, damp environment for a prolonged period – or in a situation of high wind chill and high humidity, or any scenario where more heat is lost than your body can generate. Because the signs and symptoms of hypothermia usually develop slowly and most casualties experience a gradual loss of both mental acuity and physical ability as the symptoms progress, they may not even be aware that they need emergency medical treatment.

Signs include fatigue, cold and pale skin, shivering (mild to violent), slurred speech and respiratory distress or abnormally slow breathing, confusion (including memory loss), loss of co-ordination and loss of consciousness.

In a garden context, working in the winter in wet or inadequate clothing, or falling into a pond or other cold water exposure, for example, can trigger hypothermia.

First response ✛

Hypothermia is a life-threatening condition and should always be treated as a medical emergency. It's when the shivering stops that you need to really worry as this indicates that circulation is receding and the heart is slowing. Time is of the essence. Call for help and call the emergency services. Move the casualty out of the cold. If moving him or her is not possible, add layers to insulate the casualty from further heat loss. If in wet clothes, remove what you can (within socially acceptable limits) and replace with dry clothes or wrap in dry fabric.

If the casualty becomes unconscious, layer the ground beneath him or her with a jacket or blanket and place the person into the recovery position. If he or she is not breathing and you cannot detect a pulse, commence CPR until an ambulance arrives.

Top tip

Always warm the casualty from the core/centre of the body (chest, head, neck and groin). Heat applied to the extremities (arms and legs) only forces cold blood back towards the heart and lungs, which will cause the core body temperature to drop even further – this is potentially fatal. Do not attempt to massage or rub the person vigorously if you suspect frostbite or other cold or non-cold related injuries.

CHILBLAINS

Chilblains – the medical name is perniosis – occur as a reaction to cold but not necessarily freezing temperatures. They occur more often when cold exposure is accompanied by dampness, icy water or snow – winter clearance of a pond will do it, or wrapping tender plants when it's sleeting.

Symptoms generally develop within two to fourteen hours of initial cold exposure and manifest as localised redness with swelling, often as 'skin bumps' which on re-warming of the area become tender and blue or develop itching or burning sensations. In severe cases, blisters and ulcers can form. They normally heal within a week.

Chilblains are the result of constriction damage to the capillaries and blood vessels feeding your skin and can affect hands, ears, lower legs or feet. Women gardeners are more susceptible to chilblains than men – it's nothing to do with the thickness of socks, just one of those things.

FIRST RESPONSE ✚

Warm but do not apply strong heat to the affected area to decongest blood vessels and begin natural recovery. But do this slowly, as the re-warming – the renewed blood flow – causes pain. Traditional treatment is to use steroidal cream for the itching and inflammation, and an antibiotic to ward off secondary infection. Do not scratch or burst chilblains as they can easily ulcerate. Calamine lotion or a similar lotion will ease the discomfort of itching. Ulcerated wounds need medical supervision.

GARDEN AID

A pokeweed poultice or nettle juice and/or garlic paste are folk remedies to alleviate congestion in the blood vessels. Aloe vera or juniper berry juice applied to the site will relieve itching and address secondary infections. Crambe (sea-kale) leaves are useful as an anti-itch poultice, as are acanthus leaves. Any herbal antiseptic lotion or rinse will be beneficial and the use of calamine lotion or lanolin cream can ease sensations and keep healing skin supple. Cramp bark tea or prickly ash decoctions have a history of use to remedy this condition. Undiluted lemon juice, taken internally and applied to the skin, is an old folk remedy, while the leaves of spotted laurel – used in traditional Chinese medicine and Japanese ethnobotany – are pounded to become a poultice or paste and applied to burns and chilblains and to remedy swelling. The flowers of hollyhocks are calming, while their root is soothing – both parts can form the basis of pastes, tinctures and poultices applied to ulcers and an array of skin complaints.

KITCHEN AID

Sipping a strong cup of ginger and cayenne tea, or munching a spicy snack that includes both, can help to improve circulation to the extremities.

'Ditch the Itch' Pastes

Suitable for chilblains, peeling suntan and any irritated skin conditions.

Bicarbonate of soda, cinnamon and oatmeal healer

Add 4 heaped tablespoons of bicarbonate of soda and 1 heaped tablespoon of ground cinnamon to 2 cups of finely ground oatmeal. Make a mug (2 cups) of strong camomile or linden tea and add to it 2 tablespoons of witch hazel extract. Mix all together to a porridge consistency. This will help itching, circulation and potential ulceration/infection. You can make a basinful of the mixture and soak toes for up to 30 minutes, or steep fingers in a small bowl of the healing gruel.

Lemony herbal revival

Put the antiseptic and anti-itch juice of one lemon and four sprigs each of circulatory and toxin-flushing thyme, basil, mint and lavender – discard the woody stems and just use the leaves – in a blender. Blitz and apply liberally, allowing the mixture to dry on the skin. After 20 minutes any herbage particles can be wiped off and the affected area gently washed in lukewarm water.

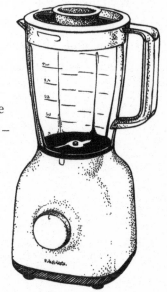

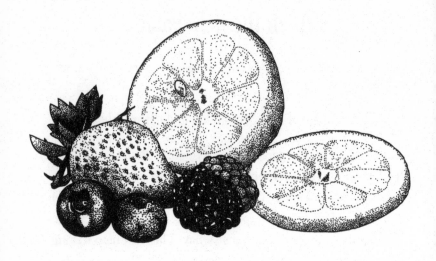

Berry blitz

Place ¼ cup of anti-itch juniper berries, ½ cup of skin revitalising strawberries and the juice of 1 cleansing lemon in a blender. Blitz and spread on the affected area. Allow to dry on the skin. After 20–30 minutes clean off and gently rinse the affected skin with salted lukewarm water.

WINTER CHEST

Exposed to the elements year round, we are all prone to the odd sniffle and cough, but being all-weather gardeners for the most part we shrug it off and perhaps have an extra glass of citrus juice or pop a cough lozenge for the vitamin C boost and the slight decongestant value.

Sometimes the sniffle becomes an all-out cold and occasionally the cough lies longer on the chest than we would like, especially in colder months when the system seems to be more susceptible to the primarily viral causes of such complaints. That said, leaky wellies and a rain-soaked back are not conducive to tip-top immunity.

Winter chest may not be an annual occurrence for gardeners who, packed with healthy fresh air, sunshine, vitamin D and the garden-gifted nutrition (if you 'grow your own'), are naturally stocked with resistance to minor illnesses, but if there is a season for chest congestion it is the winter one.

GARDEN AID

The aromatherapy of breaking a peppermint leaf releases all the decongestant menthol-like vapours that soothe and clear both congestion and the mind. And if you feel inclined to, then those same vapours can make a wonder salve to put you right if winter chest is slowing your enjoyment of the garden (see recipe on page 225). Marshmallow root and leaf tea/tincture can loosen phlegm and ease coughs, and mullein is expectorant and soothing – an oil of flower to gargle or flower tea is often the delivery method of choice.

KITCHEN AID

A quick kitchen cure is to chop some fresh ginger into boiling water and infuse for 10–20 minutes to yield a strong ginger tea, then add a teaspoon of honey to each cup as you sip throughout the day. Together, the honey and ginger assist in the loosening of mucus and soothe your throat and chest.

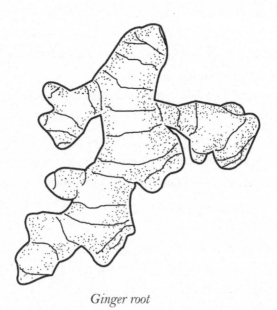

Ginger root

Mentholated Rub for Winter Chest, Coughs and Congestion

The garden yields quite a few plants that are in the ingredient list of many over-the-counter decongestant remedies, not least the aromatics that give chest rubs their unique fragrance and eye-watering potency. The secret is the menthol in the mix, which is analgesic, cooling, counter-irritant and helps to widen blood vessels – providing that 'breathe easier' sensation.

INGREDIENTS

- ½ cup sunflower oil or any alternative carrier oil
- A handful of thyme sprigs
- A handful of peppermint or other culinary mint
- A handful of eucalyptus leaves *or* 20 drops of essential oil of eucalyptus
- 10 cloves
- 25g pure beeswax
- Water to boil

YOU WILL ALSO NEED

- A saucepan
- Two glass Mason/Kilner jars or 2 Pyrex bowls
- A wooden spoon or chopstick
- Strainer/cheesecloth
- A container to store the salve

METHOD

Wash and kitchen-towel dry your herbs, then tear, crush or chop to release their active principles. Place the herbal parts and cloves into a glass jar/Pyrex bowl and cover completely with the carrier oil. Put on the lid or seal the jar/bowl. Bring a pan of water to the boil and stand the jar/bowl in the hot water and let the infusion simmer for two hours, adding water to the pan as evaporation occurs. Then turn off the heat and allow the receptacle to sit and infuse for a further 30 minutes. Now strain the herbs and cloves out of the oil, decanting it into the second jar/bowl. Chip, shave or grate the beeswax into the infused oil and stir until it dissolves fully and is mixed well. Put over a gentle heat via a bain-marie if needed. Add any essential oil at this point. Decant the mixed liquid into your storage container and allow to cool and solidify before lidding and storing for use.

The rub is intended for application by massage to the chest and back. It is suitable for inhalation and vaporising or steam bath inhalation, but is not for internal consumption. The average shelf life is approximately a year from the date it was made. Store in a cool location where it can remain semi-solid without continually re-melting and re-solidifying, thus spoiling.

HEAT RASH/PRICKLY HEAT

This is not so much an emergency as an annoyance. Heat rash or prickly heat is a red or pinkish rash occurring on areas of skin beneath clothing. It generally develops on hot days when the sweat ducts become blocked and so swell and react in rash form. The rash causes discomfort and is often itchy or prickly.

FIRST RESPONSE ✚

Heat rash is quickly remedied by removing clothing and allowing the skin to air-dry. A more persistent rash is traditionally treated with calamine lotion or a topical NSAID (non-steroidal anti-inflammatory drug), but alternatively you can take a lukewarm (or cool) bath with some bicarbonate of soda and oatmeal added to alleviate the itch. Or make a dusting powder of equal parts of bicarbonate of soda and cornflour or talcum powder to absorb the skin's moisture that is causing the heat rash, balance the body's natural pH and dissuade further reactions.

Heat rash indicates that it's time to halt gardening activities for the day and retire to a cool place before further complications such as heat cramps or heat exhaustion begin to blip at the edge of the radar. Heat rash can go as quickly as it came or take several days to resolve. For more obstinate heat rashes, a twice daily spritz of diluted vinegar acts as a skin friendly NSAID. Vinegar (acidic) and bicarbonate of soda (alkaline) cancel each other out, so don't try to combine all treatments in one go.

GARDEN AID

A decoction of magnolia bark is good against prickly heat and itching – wash the affected area in the solution. A lukewarm bath in Epsom salts or lavender luxury salts or a lukewarm shower is helpful, but a sprig of rosemary added to a vinegar bottle from a condiments set, shaken well and then applied to the skin is perhaps the most effective.

Prickly Heat Vinegar Spritz

The acetic acid in vinegar is principally a non-steroidal anti-inflammatory. White malt and apple cider vinegar both have the same active principle – you can use whatever is to hand in the larder.

METHOD

Simply dilute 50/50 some vinegar and water and decant into a bottle sprayer. Spritz the affected area twice daily. Some people experience a slight sting upon contact with the skin, but it soon dissipates and takes the itch with it.

Add some leaves of rosemary or lavender for extra cooling and soothing, and shake well before use. This will store in the fridge (with the extra bonus of the chill factor) for up to two weeks.

A sprig of rosemary in a vinegar bottle

Heat cramps

Heat cramps are muscular pains, occasionally spasms, triggered by heavy exertion and the steady loss of water and salt through excessive perspiration – a common enough garden occurrence with or without the cramp.

These cramps can take place in the abdominal muscles but most often occur in the legs or arms. They can appear as a minor tremor or just happen as a full-on event. Don't try to work through them or continue working after they dissipate. They are an indication that the day is too hot to be working and that you have been neglecting your own hydration.

First response ✚

Move to a cooler location and drink some fluid – preferably an electrolyte-containing sports drink or fruit juice with a pinch of salt, but water will do for starters.

Don't resume any strenuous activity for several hours after heat cramps have completely gone away. If cramps last longer than one hour, then medical supervision is advised.

Garden aid

Enjoy some iced mint or lemon balm tea to cool and restore, or make a healthy smoothie from your garden fruits.

Beat the Cramp Smoothie

Heat cramps are triggered by deficiencies in the electrolyte sodium. So you have to take this one both seriously and with a pinch of salt. The aim is to rehydrate and to get a blend of nutrients and mineral agents into the bloodstream and into the muscles quickly; the added salt helps that to happen and replaces the lost sodium at the same time.

INGREDIENTS

500ml unsweetened fruit juice of your choice (or whatever is in the fridge)

250ml water (or milk if you like)

Two pieces of whole fruit (fibre is good) – apple, orange, banana *or* 1 cup of garden fruits/berries.

1 teaspoon salt

Some crushed ice cubes (optional but saves time cooling the drink in the fridge)

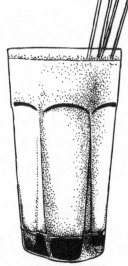

METHOD

Place all the ingredients in a blender and blitz. If using milk, it is best to blitz everything bar the milk, then add the milk and give the mixture a second whizz. Decant into a glass. Sit back, relax and enjoy your smoothie.

HEAT EXHAUSTION

Heat exhaustion is a form of shock principally triggered in gardeners by a combination of dehydration and sustained gardening activity. It manifests as heavy sweating or clammy skin with body/core temperature near normal but with a feeling of being not quite right. Pupils may dilate (widen), and headache and nausea may arise, leading to dizziness and, potentially, vomiting. It can be reversed by following the first response advice below, but it can be serious and develop further into a major medical incident.

Heat exhaustion can occur when the core temperature (the temperature inside the body) rises above the normal 37°C (98.6°F) towards 38–39°C (100–102°F) or higher.

FIRST RESPONSE

Move the casualty to a cooler location (the shade of a tree or inside a building with air conditioning). Remove some layers of clothing if the person is overdressed. Direct cooling air onto the casualty with a fan or improvised fan (folded newspaper). It is OK to sip cool, but not ice-cold, water. An isotonic drink would be helpful, but not energy drinks or caffeinated beverages. A spritz of cool water on the face and exposed skin is beneficial. A damp towel or cool compress for the head, neck or face relieves and reassures.

These methods should generally make the casualty feel much better within 15–30 minutes and without any long-term complications. But if no improvement seems to be apparent, place the casualty in the shock position (lying

231

flat on his/her back with feet raised), call an ambulance and continue to fan.

Without treatment or abatement after first aid, heat exhaustion might easily develop into heatstroke.

Heatstroke

Heatstroke is a much more serious condition than heat exhaustion. It occurs in a gardening context when heavy work on hot days, combined with inadequate rest breaks and insufficient fluid intake, forces the body into a stress reaction where it can no longer sweat or cool itself and so keeps on overheating.

With heatstroke, core temperature can rise above 40°C (104°F), at which point the cells inside the body start to break down and internal organs begin to shut down.

The symptoms of heatstroke can include a mixture of the following: feeling hot and bothered, elevated body temperature, rapid heartbeat, rapid and shallow breathing, feeling dizzy, mental confusion, headache, nausea, cessation of sweating and loss of consciousness. Untreated, it can lead to organ failure, coma, brain damage and death. Medical assistance will be required.

A key diagnostic is that heatstroke can cause the pupils of the eyes to shrink very small – to become pinned. Help the casualty to retain his/her composure and give focus to them while you await the emergency response team – for example, to count back from ten or count seconds while you check a pulse beat, or detail their movements before they became ill.

First response ⊕

Heatstroke is a medical emergency and should be treated immediately. Call for help and dial the emergency services to request an ambulance. While awaiting the arrival of the ambulance, move the casualty into a cool location (the shade of a tree or an air-conditioned room indoors). Remove layers of clothing if the person is overdressed. Direct cooling air onto the casualty with a fan or improvised fan (folded newspaper). It is OK for the casualty to sip cool, but not ice-cold, water. A spritz of cool water on the face and other exposed skin is beneficial. Wrapping in a cool, damp bed sheet will help to cool the body quickly but not so rapidly as to cause additional stress/complications.

If the casualty starts to have a seizure (fit), move nearby objects out of the way to prevent further injury. Post-fit, or if the person becomes unconscious or begins to vomit, move him or her into the recovery position and keep the airway clear. Continue to fan until the ambulance arrives.

Sunburn

Sunburn is a solar burn or more specifically a consequence of over-exposure to ultraviolet (UV) radiation emitted from the sun. It manifests as erythema (reddening) and oedema (swelling) and can be painful or hot to the touch. It can blister, peel and/or develop secondary infections, including microscopic cellular changes that pose a cancer risk (particularly of melanoma, basal cell carcinoma and squamous cell carcinoma).

In severe cases, sunburn may be considered as a second-degree burn. Sunburn in general can cause electrolyte imbalances – including dehydration – and trigger neurological stress that can result in fever, chills, fainting and even circulatory shock.

First response

Remove yourself/the casualty from further damage – get inside or into shade. Rehydrate and fan the areas of hot skin. A cool to lukewarm shower or bath can ease side-effects, but do not cool too rapidly. Leave blisters intact – if they burst on their own then apply an antibacterial wash or ointment. The main treatment is to provide relief to the discomfort of the burn – generally with analgesics or 'after sun' skin moisturisers.

Garden aid

Prevention is better than cure, so on sunny days try to avoid sun exposure between 10 a.m. and 2 p.m. Note that the shade of a tree in full leaf can provide sun protection to around 10–20 SPF but you will need more than that to shield your skin. Wear suitable protective clothing including long sleeves, sunglasses, wide-brimmed hats and apply a sun block with a factor of at least 30+ SPF regularly (not just once!).

Succulents, notably aloe vera, can provide a cooling sap which, as well as the cooling effect, lessens the reddening and triggers skin regeneration. Many herbal teas can reduce inflammation and will help with their calming influence as well as their other properties. If chilled, many can be spritzed onto hot skin for post-sun relief. Crambe and acanthus leaves can be blended with natural yoghurt or steamed and cooled to make a poultice with the benefit of their anti-itch, astringent, cleansing and emollient properties.

KITCHEN AID

The dairy fats in milk and yoghurts are good for UV radiation damage and cooling too, when applied topically. Try a squeeze of lemon juice or a dash of apple cider vinegar to cool, reduce inflammation, disinfect and promote faster recovery.

After-sun Remedies

Quick-fix after-sun soother

Bicarbonate of soda helps to balance your skin's pH and speed recovery/ healing. Black tea has tannins to reduce inflammation and promote healing. Natural yoghurt is a cooling agent but also, like bicarbonate of soda, works to adjust the pH of skin and triggers faster healing with natural enzymes to speed sunburn recovery.

In a cup, moisten 2 tablespoons of black or green tea (or two opened tea bags) with 2–3 tablespoons of boiling water. Let it rest for 1 minute, then add 2 tablespoons of bicarbonate of soda and stir in a dollop of natural yoghurt. Stir well and apply to the hot skin. Store in the fridge for up to three days and apply often to cool and remedy.

Quick-fix after-sun peel-heal gel

The sap of a leaf of aloe vera mixed with 1–2 tablespoons of vinegar can slow or prevent peeling, with the bonus of providing a cooling sensation. To boost the gel's healing properties you can grate in a few slices of cucumber or some raw potato flesh and blitz in a blender with 20 drops of lavender essential oil.

Garden after-sun lotion

Boil five fingers of washed comfrey root (an anti-inflammatory) in ½ cup of water and turn off the heat. Add 1 tablespoon of zinc ointment, then 3 tablespoons of skin-softening liquid lecithin or 1 tablespoon of honey, 2 tablespoons of cocoa or shea butter and 3 tablespoons of almond/olive oil. Blend all to a pulp. Add 10 drops each of lavender, tea tree and orange (or bergamot) essential oils. This has a shelf life of three months if stored in the refrigerator.

JUST ONE OF THOSE THINGS

Here I cover those events not necessarily accidental but none the less injurious: dehydration from over-working without a tea break or two; or things like hyperventilation, such as might occur with a panicking casualty. And emotional shock can accompany any garden mishap. They are the 'just one of those things' types of event that could be featured in other sections of the book but fit equally well gathered conveniently into one place here.

HYPERVENTILATION

Hyperventilation can accompany any accident. It is the panic response triggering respiratory distress and manifests as fast, excessively deep breathing and can progress to a full-blown panic attack or dissipate as quickly as it came. It can be a side-effect of shock. It can also present with dizziness, feeling faint and a limb trembling scenario first, with a noticeable tingling in the hands or feet.

FIRST RESPONSE ⊕

Reassurance and resituating are the watchwords of treatment. Offer firm but kind reassurance that 'everything will be all right', 'it will pass', 'try to relax', 'take slow breaths', etc. Removing the casualty from the cause of distress is another aid to recovery.

If the panic is part of a more serious injury (blood loss,

severed finger, etc.) then assure the casualty that all is under control. If the injury triggering panic is severe, call for an ambulance and prepare to tackle both shock and the causative injury.

Do not use the 'paper bag trick' – breathing into a paper bag – as new research now suggests that this does not help; instead, help the casualty to breathe fresh air.

Focus calms, so get the casualty to count the duration of each breath, to follow the second hand on a wristwatch or a stopwatch feature on a mobile phone – time each inhalation to last for seven seconds and each exhalation for eleven seconds. Count with the casualty if necessary. After a minute of this, normal breathing patterns should return. If not, and the casualty is still unwell, medical assistance is required to rule out other causes (such as poisoning, etc.).

Dehydration

Dehydration is what happens when your body loses more fluid than you take in. It is an ever-present threat when under the influence of gardening activities, even on days not forecast as having heatwave temperatures. You can perspire just as easily mowing the lawn or digging a bed over on a cool day as you can in mid-July.

Dehydration is more than a strong thirst, though that is one of the symptoms, alongside tiredness, light-headedness and dark, odorous urine. Dehydration is a disruption of the body's natural balance. Water makes up over two-thirds of a normal healthily functioning human body; it is intrinsic on a cellular level to all organs and their functions but when the natural water balance of the body is reduced it also disrupts the delicate balance of electrolyte salts (especially sodium and potassium) and blood sugars (glucose), which further disrupts functions, including the capacity to think clearly.

If left untreated dehydration soon becomes severe and leads to seizures, brain damage and even death.

First response ✛

Drink plenty of fluids – water, diluted squash and fruit juice are all recommended but it is best to avoid fizzy drinks and caffeine. If symptoms persist or the casualty manifests rapid heartbeat, strong fatigue, an inability to pass urine after rehydrating, or feeling quite unwell, then medical supervision is required.

GARDEN AID

Sit in/place the casualty in the shade. Spritz/splash some water from a hose onto the face and neck. Pinch some mint or lemon balm for a quick, rejuvenating inhale and then drop the leaves into a glass of iced water.

Quick-fix Isotonic Drinks

Isotonic drinks are designed to quickly replace the fluids that are lost by exertion and perspiration. They beat water through having a supply of carbohydrates/sugars to replenish energy. The trick is in the salt – as sodium is the electrolyte lost most readily in perspiration, adding it to drinks makes the fluid more isosmotic. This means that it brings the drink closer to the same concentration of solutes as the blood and so is more readily absorbed into the bloodstream – perfect to offset the physiological reactions to dehydration. But they don't have to be store-bought. I prefer mine to be homemade.

Juicy version

Place the following ingredients in a jug and stir.

500ml fruit juice (whatever you have handy)

500ml still water

Pinch of salt

Pinch of sugar

Ice (optional)

Squish squash version

Place the following ingredients in a jug and stir.

200ml concentrated fruit squash (often high in glucose)

800ml still water

A squeeze of fresh lime, lemon or orange juice

Pinch of salt

Ice (optional)

EMOTIONAL SHOCK

Emotional shock is the state of distress that accompanies any calamity/accident. It can be severe if the accident was/is severe (severed body part, etc.) and so can become more of a psychological trauma (often manifesting post-event). Counselling and the support of loved ones is vital in recovery from incidents of that scale.

On the bottom rung of the ladder, the emotional shock that could accompany most of the accidents and ailments listed in this book are mild distress, perturbation, distraction or disbelief, accompanied by a little adrenaline, a little embarrassment and maybe even an angry outburst or internal feelings of guilt. Once you have dusted off the seat of your pants, bandaged your finger, cussed out the rake handle or iced your toe, then a cup of tea or hot chocolate is as good as a hug – and will counter those fizzing neurotransmitters and endorphins that arise from panic, being shocked, getting angry or being a little shaken up. A cup of daylily flower tea is considered to be anodyne and antispasmodic, and I find it somewhat sedative. Traditionally used in parts of China to manage childbirth, it adds a nuance to camomile when the chill factor is urgently called for.

But chocolate, with all that oxytocin, is the best in my book and so I think it is nice and fitting to end the injury chapter with a cake recipe. Yes, I said cake – the final remedy/recipe being a big sweet kiss of blissful chocolate cake to get the right endorphins and neurotransmitters singing – excellent with that badly needed cup of tea or mug of hot chocolate. It is obviously not for you or your casualty if the emotional shock is part of an accident that means nil by mouth until medical invention is ruled out or concluded – but worth the wait when you can get round to it in recovery. And to the rest – they say a change is as good as a rest, and certainly the only thing that beats a day of gardening is a day of baking ... or a night of passion, and chocolate is good for that too – win–win all the way!!

A Big Sweet Kiss of Blissful Chocolate Cake

Makes an 8 inch/20cm square cake for slicing or a single 9 inch/22cm round cake for gluttonising.

INGREDIENTS FOR THE CAKE

1 cup brewed coffee *or* chicory substitute

1 large cooked beetroot (definitely *not* the pickled variety)

2 cups plain white flour

½ cup cocoa powder *or* drinking chocolate

½ cup chocolate, grated or broken

2 teaspoons brown sugar *or* Stevia sugar substitute

1 heaped teaspoon bicarbonate of soda

½ teaspoon salt

¾ cup almond butter *or* ½ cup vegetable oil

3 tablespoons honey

1 tablespoon apple cider vinegar

FOR THE GANACHE TOPPING

300g good quality chocolate, broken into pieces

300ml double cream

METHOD

Preheat the oven to 190°C/375°F/Gas Mark 5. Line the cake tin with baking parchment or greaseproof paper.

Make a cup of coffee or chicory with hot water.

Purée the cooked beetroot – use a little of the coffee/chicory liquid to get a start if needed.

Sift all the dry ingredients into a large mixing bowl. Add the coffee and other wet ingredients (butter/oil, honey, beetroot purée, etc.) except for the vinegar. Mix all to a smoothish batter – the grated/chipped chocolate will be lumpy for now.

Next add the vinegar and give a quick stir through. Expect pale swirls where the vinegar is reacting with the bicarbonate of soda in the mix – this is the body/rise to your cake – all good.

Lastly, pour the batter into the prepared baking tin and bake for 35 minutes.

Once cooked through, you can set the cake aside to cool and then glaze with the ganache, or serve it warm with the ganache as a sauce.

To make the ganache

While the cake is baking, heat a saucepan of water until boiling, for the bain-marie.

Break up the chocolate.

Place a bowl over the hot water in the saucepan (but not touching the surface of the water), add the chocolate fragments and stir to melt. Once the chocolate has melted, remove from the heat and fold in the cream, stirring until smooth.

Once the mixture is smooth and has cooled, pipe or spoon it over your cake.

PS: 'Gan' in Irish means 'without', and this ganache-topped cake may just leave you without those aches and pains. That said, if you burn a fingertip in the process of making the cake, see page 122!

FIRST AID
CORE SKILLS

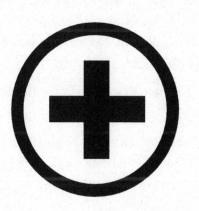

In this section the skills and techniques universally applied by first aiders are detailed. They will support the advice already given in some of the earlier entries, and will upgrade your skills to deal with more serious matters than just splinters or stings. While this book is predominately about garden aid, there is no harm at all in having some proficiency in first aid.

THE FIRST STEPS OF FIRST AID (DR-ABC)

- **D**anger – make sure it is safe for you to proceed. Check there is no spreading fire, chemical fumes, live wires, etc.

- **R**esponse – what is the casualty's state – conscious, unconscious, dazed, in shock? Can he or she hear you? Can the casualty speak, blink and make movements? Does he or she respond to touch?

- **A**irway – check for a blockage in the throat – an object or lolling tongue.

- **B**reathing – once the airway is cleared, if the casualty cannot breathe easily it may indicate shock or respiratory distress and the need for rescue breathing and eventual CPR. Place your ear close to the casualty's mouth and nose to listen for breath sounds and detect air/moisture from the breath. Look at the casualty's chest for signs of movement.

- **C**irculation – is there a pulse? If there is, is it weak/strong/racing? If it is non-existent, proceed immediately with CPR.

ESTABLISHING AN AIRWAY

With unconscious casualties, the tongue is the most common cause of airway obstruction. The tongue is not 'swallowed' but rather has slipped/lolled to a lower position that blocks the pharynx and the airway passage. By repositioning the lower jaw to a forward position the tongue is lifted away from the back of the throat and clears the airway. Establishing an airway should take a matter of seconds.

HEAD-TILT/CHIN-LIFT METHOD

This is the preferred option where a neck fracture is not suspected.

1. Kneel beside the casualty's head/shoulders.
2. Place a hand on the casualty's forehead.
3. With the palm of your hand apply firm, backward pressure – encouraging the casualty's head to tilt back.
4. With your other hand, place your fingertips under the bony protrusion of the casualty's chin.
5. Lift the chin with your fingertips until the upper and lower teeth are almost brought together but with the mouth still open.

JAW-THRUST METHOD

A technique to move the casualty's tongue forward without extending the neck – for cases of suspected neck fracture.

1. Kneel behind the casualty's head.

2. Allow your elbows to anchor/rest on the surface on which the casualty is lying.

3. Position a hand on each side of the casualty's head.

4. Position the tips of your index and middle fingers under the angles of the jaw – keeping one hand on either side of the jaw.

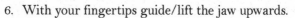

5. Position your thumbs just below the level of the teeth – to steady the casualty's head and prevent turning or tilting during the lift manoeuvre.

6. With your fingertips guide/lift the jaw upwards.

7. The mouth should be open, not closed. If necessary use a thumb to retract the casualty's lower lip.

If the jaw-thrust method does not quickly establish an airway then guide/lift the jaw up a little further to better reposition the tongue. If the additional lift is still unsuccessful, sweep mouth with a finger. If there is still no result, proceed to the head-tilt/chin-lift method above – it is considered in EMS, mountain rescue, etc., that in the survival of a casualty the importance of maintaining an airway outweighs the risk of suspected spinal injury.

CHECK FOR BREATHING – FOUR WAYS TO ASCERTAIN RESPIRATION

1. Lung activity/chest movement – look for the rise and fall of the chest.

2. Audible sounds – listen for the sound of regular inhalations and exhalations; gasps and rattles do not indicate a clear airway.

3. Breathed air sensation – place your ear close to the mouth and nose to detect air flow.

4. Breath moisture – use a mirror to check for condensation of the breath.

RESCUE BREATHING

This is the technique of breathing for an unconscious casualty who is not breathing for him/herself, but has a pulse. (If there is no pulse, proceed immediately to CPR.) Once an airway is established the casualty is in a position to receive rescue breathing, but there is a slight variance in approach between adult and child casualties so both are outlined here. While mouth-to-mouth is no longer universally applied because of contagious diseases and contemporary sensibilities, it is a skill I personally value knowing – in case a loved one of mine ever needs it.

RESCUE BREATHING FOR AN ADULT CASUALTY

1. Establish an airway.

2. Use a resuscitation mask if available, or a barrier against potential contagious disease.

3. Gently pinch the casualty's nose shut.

4. Place/seal your mouth over the casualty's open mouth.

5. Breathe a breath slowly into the casualty's mouth/lungs.

6. Watch to see the chest rise. (If chest does not rise and fall, try re-establishing the airway again.)

7. Take a breath and repeat numbers 5 and 6. (If still no rise and fall, proceed to abdominal thrusts, see page 263.)

8. Give one breath every 5 seconds. (Don't pump up the lungs with quick successions of breaths; rather, pause between each rescue breath to let the air flow out. It is helpful to count the seconds as 'one–one thousand, two–one thousand' etc.)

9. After two rescue breaths, check for a pulse. If a pulse is present continue the rescue breathing for a further minute (12 breaths).

10. Check pulse again; if present, continue rescue breathing until the ambulance arrives. If no pulse, proceed to CPR.

RESCUE BREATHING FOR AN INFANT OR CHILD BELOW THE AGE OF TEN

Because the first few minutes are crucial to prevent brain damage, with an infant or child it is recommended that you give rescue breaths for a minute even before you call the emergency services. I recommend you call out for help while attending to the child or dial 999 or 112 on a speakerphone before beginning life-saving techniques – you can tell the operator your location and type of emergency between breaths.

1. Establish an airway with a slight tilt – the angle required is less for a child.

2. Pinch the nose closed, place/seal your mouth over the casualty's open mouth (*and* nose if it is an infant).

3. Follow instructions 5–10 as for an adult, giving one breath every 3 rather than every 5 seconds.

HOW TO TAKE A PULSE

The pulse is an indication of circulation; it is used to check blood flow to a limb, non-constriction of bandages or casts and as a prime means of detecting a heartbeat. Where the heartbeat is being monitored, if you are having difficulty detecting a pulse at one location, try a second point to make sure.

The pulse of a casualty can be found where an artery passes close to the skin and is easily checked using the fingers. Never use your thumb to take a pulse as it has a pulse of its own. The prime points for checking the pulse include the neck and wrist.

THE WRIST/RADIAL ARTERY

1. Extend the casualty's hand with palm facing upwards and elbow slightly bent.
2. Position your index and middle finger close together below the wrist crease.
3. Press down lightly and feel for the beat.

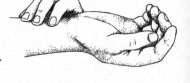

If you can't feel a pulse at the wrist or the wrist is burnt, bleeding or otherwise unreliable, then try the carotid artery.

THE NECK/CAROTID ARTERY

This is located on the side of the neck below the ear/jaw and easily checked with the index and middle fingers. The carotid artery pulses can be detected in the hollow below the jaw and towards the ear – there are subtle variations, but this is a handy landmark.

ALTERNATIVE PULSE POINTS (ALSO PRESSURE POINTS FOR BLEEDING CONTROL)

Use to check circulation with bandaging, crush injuries or in cases where traditional points are burnt, damaged or otherwise inaccessible.

- The dorsalis pedis – on the arch at the top of the foot (located between the first and second metatarsal bones).

- The posterior tibial artery – the ankle joint.

- The popliteal artery – behind the knee.

- The brachial artery – inside the elbow or just under the biceps.

- The femoral artery – in the groin.

- The abdominal aorta – over the abdomen.

- The apex of the heart – in the chest.

- The superficial temporal artery – in the temple.

- The basilar artery – close to the ear.

LISTENING TO THE HEARTBEAT

A heartbeat indicates life. The various rates indicate conditions: fast equals panic, slow equals shock, etc. It is measured in beats per minute (bpm) – the beats are counted for a timed minute and the 'normal' rate varies with age:

- Babies up to 1 year: 100–160 bpm.
- Children aged 1–10 years: 60–140 bpm.
- Children aged 10+ and adolescents: 60–100 bpm.
- Adults: 60–100 bpm.

Traditionally the beats are counted out over a timed minute, but in an emergency assessment you can count the beats over a 20-second period and then multiply the beat total by 3 to supply a guide/indication rate.

How to Listen to a Heartbeat

When the body goes into shutdown, the pulse may be so weak it is hard to find, but a heartbeat might be more discernible.

- For men: Place your ear just below the breastbone, slightly to the left of the right nipple.
- For women: Place your ear below the right breast.
- For children: Place your ear a little to the left of the right nipple.

(All left/right body descriptions are as seen by you facing the casualty.)

CARDIOPULMONARY RESUSCITATION (CPR)

CPR is a technique to revive circulation and keep blood and oxygen moving around the body by manually fibrillating or pumping the heart externally.

CHEST COMPRESSION — HANDS-ONLY CPR

If you have not previously been trained in CPR or are worried about giving mouth-to-mouth resuscitation to an unknown person, then chest compressions or hands-only CPR is ideal.

1. Establish an airway.
2. Place the heel of the hand on the breastbone at the centre of the chest.
3. Place the other hand on top of the first.
4. Interlock fingers or grip comfortably for sustained compressions.

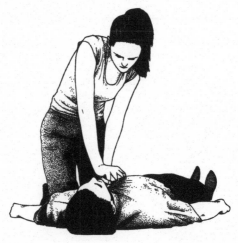

5. Carry out the compressions – pressing straight down.

6. Repeat the compressions at a rate mimicking the heartbeat (see *Top tip*).

7. Continue the compressions until the ambulance arrives or you can no longer continue.

Top tip

When compressing, use the weight of your body, not just your arms. Press straight down, by 5–6cm (around 2in) on the chest and release before repeating the compression. This movement mimics the beat of the heart. It can be carried out to the rhythm of the song 'Stayin' Alive' by the Bee Gees, or around 100 compressions per minute.

CPR WITH RESCUE BREATHS

ADULT CPR

1. Airway to compression (numbers 1 to 5 in the above list).

2. After every thirty chest compressions, seal your mouth over the casualty's mouth – exhale/blow inward to inflate their lungs. Watch for the chest to rise, so that you can detect any blockage and/or know if the CPR is working.

3. Give two rescue breaths, each over one second long, then return to a second set of thirty compressions before administering two more breaths.

4. Continue with cycles of thirty chest compressions and two rescue breaths until the ambulance arrives or the casualty revives.

CHILD CPR

With infants and children under 10 years of age, if deprived of oxygen (not breathing), permanent brain damage can occur within 4 minutes and death can occur after 4–6 minutes, so it is vital to act quickly and maintain CPR until the child can breathe by him/herself or until the emergency services take over. Having patted the child's back (if there is no danger of neck or back injury), cleared the airway and given initial rescue breaths, begin child CPR.

The CPR procedure is modified for children in the following manner: to perform chest compressions, first place one hand on the child's forehead to tilt the head back and open the airway, place the heel of the other hand on the child's breastbone (just below the nipples – not at the very lowest part of the breastbone) and press down so that the chest compresses to about a third to half the depth of the chest and then let the chest rise completely. Give thirty of these chest compressions in rapid succession – no pauses. If breathing has not resumed after that, then cover the child's mouth tightly with yours. Pinch the nose closed; with a small infant, your mouth will seal/cover the nose. Keeping the casualty's chin lifted and head tilted, give two rescue breaths, each of one second duration – the chest will rise. Resume thirty compressions as before, then give another two rescue breaths. Continue this cycle until help arrives or the child recovers. If recovery occurs before the emergency services arrive, place the child in the recovery position and monitor him or her.

USING A DEFIBRILLATOR/AED (AUTOMATED EXTERNAL DEFIBRILLATOR) DEVICE

AEDs are automated, so you just follow their lead – they will analyse the casualty's heart rhythm several times to be certain it is in a 'shockable' rhythm before asking you to proceed. AEDs have instructions printed on them, but in general these are:

1. Turn on the AED.

2. Wipe the casualty's chest to ensure it is dry.

3. Position and attach the pads.

4. Make sure no one is touching the casualty.

5. Push the 'Analyse' button.

6. If a shock is advised, clear and push the 'Shock' button.

7. After the shock has finished, follow the AED prompts.

8. There is no live current to the body at this point, so it is safe to start/resume CPR and chest compressions.

RECOVERY POSITIONS

In situations where a casualty is unconscious but breathing and with no apparent other life-threatening conditions, placing the person in a recovery position ensures an open airway, prevents choking and stabilises the body until an ambulance arrives. It is also sometimes used to rest or provide a calming opportunity for a conscious casualty while awaiting an ambulance or other support.

THE TRADITIONAL RECOVERY POSITION – A LYING DOWN RECOVERY POSITION

1. Kneel beside the casualty.

2. Place the nearest arm to you at a right angle to his/her body, with the palm upwards.

3. Take the casualty's other hand and place the back of it against the cheek nearest you to steady the head in readiness for rolling over – this will also support the casualty's head when he or she is turned.

4. Reach across to the casualty's leg that is furthest from you, and reposition so that the leg is bent with the foot flat on the floor.

5. Gently pull that leg/knee towards you so that the casualty slowly rolls over onto his/her side.

6. Use this bent knee to stabilise the casualty's position.

7. Check the airway is clear.

8. Monitor breathing and pulse until the ambulance arrives.

RECOVERY POSITION FOR HEART ATTACK – THE W-POSITION

This is often called the W-position but can appear more like an italic *N*: with the casualty sitting on the ground, with feet on the ground, knees bent and shoulders supported – think of the right vertical stroke of the *N* as the casualty's back, the left vertical stroke as the shin and feet and the diagonal line as the thigh part of the leg from knee to buttocks. From this *N* you can angle the casualty back into a looser, more comfortable slant/lean and let their feet just rest gently out – transforming the *N* into a sort of W. Either way, this half sitting, half leaning back position is best to maintain a comfortable breathing rhythm and sense of control.

RECOVERY POSITION FOR SHOCK

Place the casualty flat on his/her back and raise the feet above the level of the heart.

POSSIBLE SPINAL INJURY

Moving the casualty in cases of suspected spinal injury can cause further serious injury and is not recommended unless the casualty is vomiting, choking or in a situation of further danger or injury. If, however, it is necessary, moving the casualty is best carried out by a two-person team. One person should take up a position at the head of the casualty and another alongside his/her body. Working together, carefully roll the casualty onto one side – while keeping his/her head, neck and back aligned (a jacket or cushion may help to frame and support the neck and head) – but do not tilt the head or take it out of alignment.

RECOVERY POSITION FOR BABIES LESS THAN A YEAR OLD

Cradle the baby in your arms but with its head tilted downwards to keep the airway open.

COPING WITH CHOKING

ABDOMINAL THRUSTS AND THE HEIMLICH MANOEUVRE

For cases of choking or airway obstruction by a swallowed object, the aim is to increase airway pressure behind the obstructing object, thus forcing its ejection from the windpipe. The Heimlich technique can be used on adults and children over one year old; it will need to be modified for babies and pregnant women.

PRE-THRUST BACK SLAP

Sometimes a firm slap/blow between the shoulder blades with the palm/heel of the hand is enough to dislodge the blockage. Have the casualty lean forward and give five such back blows. If this is not effective, then go on to Heimlich thrusts.

HEIMLICH THRUSTS

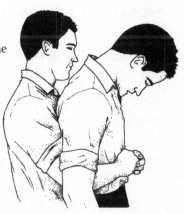

1. Position yourself behind the casualty.

2. Reach your arms around his/her waist.

3. Bring the hands together, making a fist of the hand closest to the casualty's body.

4. Position the fist, with thumb side in, just above the person's navel at the bottom of the rib cage.

5. Grip the fist tightly with the other hand.

6. Pull the fist abruptly inward and upward.

HEIMLICH GROUND THRUSTS

If the person is conscious and lying on his or her back but cannot be lifted because of injury, straddle the person, facing their head. Place the heel of one hand just above the navel at the bottom of the ribcage, place the other hand on top and press with a quick upper thrust.

HEIMLICH MANOEUVRE FOR A PREGNANT WOMAN

To protect the unborn baby it is best to position your hands a little higher than normal. Reposition the fist to the base of the breastbone, just above the point where the lowest ribs join.

HEIMLICH MANOEUVRE ON ONESELF

Option A: Make a fist. Place the thumb of it below your rib cage, above your navel. Grasp the fist with your other hand and pull it into you with a quick upward movement.

Option B: Lean over the back of a chair, a table edge or even a railing and thrust your upper abdomen against that edge.

ABDOMINAL THRUSTS ON A BABY UP TO ONE YEAR OLD

DISLODGING

Sit down and rest your forearm on your thigh so that you can hold the baby face-down supported by your forearm (carefully support the head with your palm). Gravity may dislodge the object, but if not give the baby five gentle but firm back thumps.

BABY THRUSTS

If dislodgement fails then turn the baby over – face-up on your forearm – with head lower than the body. Place your index and middle fingers just below the baby's breastbone and carry out five quick chest thrusts. Repeat cycles of back blows and thrusts until the object is dislodged.

THE UNCONSCIOUS CASUALTY

When a casualty becomes unconscious, muscles relax and if he or she is lying on his/her back then the tongue can easily fall back into the throat and impede air flow. If safe to do so (no spinal injury or wound complications), turning the casualty into the recovery position and sweeping the mouth to reposition the tongue and to check for other obstructions is traditional practice. Dial the emergency services and keep the casualty protected, monitoring vital signs until an ambulance arrives. Administer CPR if the casualty stops breathing.

STOPPING BLEEDING

Stopping bleeding is a prime concern in first aid and there are various techniques depending on the nature of the wound and the intensity of the bleed – more detail is given under entries for bleeding and wounds (see page 112ff). The general rule is to apply direct pressure – the weight of a firmly placed hand, adhesive plaster or a dressing is often enough to stem the flow and allow the wound to clot within minutes, or to hold back further loss until an ambulance arrives. At other times a pressure point technique will be required to put pressure on the vein supplying blood to the open wound.

DIRECT PRESSURE

Sometimes all you have available is your hand, but the sleeve of a shirt or t-shirt can act as a barrier when applying manual direct pressure – hold the wound but do not squeeze, and apply downward pressure to stem the flow. Most minor wounds will clot after 10–15 minutes of such pressure. With major bleeds, the objective is to stem as much blood loss as possible until the ambulance arrives.

PRESSURE POINT TECHNIQUE

If blood flow has not been halted within 20 minutes of direct pressure and a dressing you are likely to be in the realms of blood vessel damage. In this case, dial the emergency services if that has not already been done. You may need to put pressure on the nearest main artery supplying blood to the area. If blood is spurting out you will definitely and instantly need to press down on that artery, firmly against the bone, to cut off the supply until the emergency services arrive.

LAST RESORT TOURNIQUET TECHNIQUE

I say 'last resort' as many a good limb has been lost to the panicky application of a tourniquet – an ambulance generally arrives quite promptly but the damage could be done before professional help arrives. Pressure points and elevation will generally stem enough of the flow without killing the circulation. That said, however, as a last resort when all else fails and loss of life is imminent, then tourniquets can save the life of the injured person – whether or not the limb can be saved. If needs must, then the best way to proceed is as follows:

1. Use a t-shirt, shirt sleeve or a big enough piece of cloth at least 5–6cm (2in) wide to wrap around an extremity like a bandage.

2. Place the tourniquet several inches to a hand's width above the site of the injury towards the heart, or above the affected joint.

3. Tie as needed to stop it slipping from its position.

4. Using a stick, pencil or other rigid object as a torsion device, slide it through the wrapped cloth.

5. Twist the torsion object to tighten the bandage until it completely cuts off circulation.

6. Tie the ends of the bandage to the torsion device to stop it unwinding.

7. Always note the time at which you first tightened the tourniquet. This information will help the emergency services assess the side-effects of potential blood flow restriction.

WOUND CLEANSING AND DRESSING

WOUND CLEANSING – INITIAL WOUND

With bleeding controlled, an open wound can be cleansed gently with mild soap and water, a saline solution or an antiseptic solution (homemade or commercial). Sometimes cleaning an open wound can cause bleeding to re-start – usually in a minor manner. Stem the flow again with direct pressure and then proceed with applying the dressing.

WOUND CLEANSING – WOUND CARE

Wound cleansing as a care regime for wounds in recovery is a complicated issue, perennially picked over – the preferred techniques of wound cleansing have always moved with the times: the most ancient practice of honey bandages is currently back in favour and antiseptic swabbing is under revision as potentially being damaging to the natural healing processes of tissue. It has long been understood that bactericides and other constituents present in wound exudate stimulate the inflammatory response, but the understanding now is that the inflammation naturally results in improved blood supply to the wound site and with it the delivery of white blood cell neutrophils and macrophages which ingest bacteria naturally. Keeping the wound clean and moist is the best you can do for it, but over-enthusiastic cleansing can impede healing unless the wound is clinically infected. Ask advice from your doctor for your particular wound and its required care regime.

WOUND DRESSING

Wounds come in all shapes and sizes and each type will require different management and treatment procedures during the various stages of healing, so there is no 'one size fits all' dressing, but there are common objectives:

- Be sterile and non-toxic.

- Protect the wound from contamination without sticking to, shedding fibres into, or generally causing additional trauma to the wound on application or by later removal.

- Cover the wound completely.

- Maintain a moist (not wet) environment at the wound site, as this is conducive to healing.

- Assist with the management/control of excess exudate.

- Help to stabilise/immobilise an injured area but do not interfere unnecessarily with movement and other body functions.

BANDAGING TECHNIQUES

- A bandage should be applied firmly but not tightly.

- Work from the side of the affected part to avoid reaching across the casualty or into the injury zone.

- Affected parts may swell post-bandaging, so monitor regularly to check whether the bandage needs to be loosened or re-tied.

- When bandaging an arm or leg, aim to leave fingers/toes exposed to check circulation.

- Elbows and knees are best bandaged in a slightly bent position.

- The two most common bandaging techniques are the spiral method and the figure-of-eight (see below).

SPIRAL TECHNIQUE

This is best employed to wrap cylindrical parts of the body, such as the lower leg and the forearm.

1. Start below the wound.
2. Apply two turns in a circular motion to secure the starting point.
3. Wind the bandage upwards in a spiral fashion, with each overlap a third to a half of the bandage's diameter, to completely cover and secure the wound site.
4. Finish with a two circular turns and secure with tape or a safety pin.

FIGURE-OF-EIGHT TECHNIQUE

This is best employed to wrap joints – elbows and knees, for example – and to secure dressings in place.

1. Flex the joint and begin with two straight turns to wrap the joint.
2. Working away from the body, make figure-of-eight turns, above and below the joint.
3. Continue to wind the bandage in this fashion, with each overlap a third to a half of the bandage's diameter, to completely cover and secure the wound site.
4. Finish with a two circular turns and secure with adhesive tape or a safety pin.

MAKING A SLING

1. Cut or diagonally fold a piece of cloth to form a triangle.

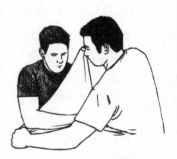

2. Have the elbow of the injured arm bent at a right angle, resting on the chest.

3. Slip one end of the triangle up under the injured arm and over the opposite shoulder.

4. Bring the dangling end of the triangle up towards the shoulder of the injured arm. The sling will naturally take shape and the injured arm will now be inside the triangle, with the elbow covered at one end and fingers peeking out at the other.

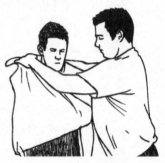

5. Adjust the sling so that the hand is higher than the elbow, to maintain circulation and decrease pain.

6. Tie the top ends together at the side (*not* the back) of the neck on the uninjured side.

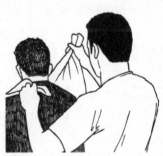

7. Take the remaining corner point of the triangle – at the elbow – and with a safety pin attach it to the sling. Or as an alternative twist the point and tie it off.

8. Slip some padding under the knot at the shoulder for comfort.

COLLAR AND CUFF SLING

This kind of sling is used when a suspected fracture of the collarbone or elbow complicates sling adjustments, or when a triangular sling is not available.

A single torn-off strip of cloth, shirt sleeve, nylon tights or a trouser belt can be made into a collar and cuff sling: simply place the length of fabric under the cuff (wrist) and tie off at the collar (neck). This simple strap will support the weight of the limb and immobilise any injury until medical help arrives.

MAKING A SPLINT

A splint is a rigid support structure to immobilise an injury to prevent further damage and to decrease pain. It is important to stop any bleeding and care for any wounds before applying a splint. Injured body parts are usually splinted in the position in which they are found – realignment should be done by the emergency services. In some circumstances an injured body part can be taped to an uninjured body part – e.g. toe to toe – but for the most part a framework is built around the injury to secure it. If the injury is more painful after splinting, then loosen or remove the splint completely.

1. Source something rigid to use as a support framework – a stick, garden stake, a rolled-up magazine.

2. Select a length that will extend the splint beyond the injured area for complete immobilisation.

3. Aim to include the joint above and below the injury within the splint structure.

4. Aim to pad the injury/splint interface to avoid putting extra pressure on the damaged limb.

5. Once positioned and constructed, secure the rigid structures of the splint using adhesive tape, garden ties, a belt, etc.

6. Secure above and below the injury.

7. Check the circulation and that the splint is not too tight.

RECOGNISING A FRACTURE

The casualty may feel the break or even hear a snap but sometimes nobody is quite sure whether it is a break. There is often extreme pain but we all have different pain tolerances so it is better to diagnose by checking the following:

1. Is there a grating sound when the limb is moved?

2. Is there partial or complete loss of motion?

3. Is there deformity or abnormal motion at the fracture site?

4. Is there swelling, pain with muscle spasms, tingling or numbness?

If the answer is yes to any of these questions, it means there is a fracture.

TREATING A BURN

Most minor burns can be treated at home and perhaps with a follow-up GP appointment, but major burns instigate circulatory shock, so call the emergency services promptly.

1. Cool the burn immediately with flowing cool/tepid water – hold an arm under the tap/knee under a shower head, for example.

2. Irrigate for 20 minutes.

3. Remove rings from burnt hands and potential constrictions from other body parts before swelling begins.

4. Cover the burn. Using strips of cling film (layered on the burn, not wrapped around) is ideal as it will not stick to the wound – alternatively use a damp cloth or tea towel – this will continue to cool and protect the wound.

5. Anything greater than a minor scald or finger burn may require tetanus treatment and medical intervention (including plastic surgery or scar minimisation) so take the casualty to a doctor or the emergency room at the hospital.

Top tips

Do not apply butter, oils or greasy substances to fresh burns. Do not apply adhesive, sticky or fluffy dressings. Do not prick or pick at blisters.

Flushing eyes

You may just need to wash out some grit or the splash of a homemade liquid feed, or it might be a more serious chemical splash. Even with seemingly minor incidents, if there is still irritation or any vision loss after flushing the eyes then take the casualty to hospital for professional medical treatment. For major events, always see flushing as a pre-treatment (like cooling a burn) before you get to the emergency room.

1. Rinse eye(s) with a clean source of water – from a tap or garden hose.

2. Keep the eye(s) open at all times during the rinse.

3. Flush eye(s) for at least 20 minutes.

4. Assess the situation – do you need further medical support?

Top tips

If using a flowing tap, position the casualty's head so that the affected eye is lower than the unaffected one. If using a garden hose, hold it vertically so that the water bubbles straight up rather than applying jet pressure to the eye.

ASSESSING THE NEED FOR STITCHES

Three simple questions will decide whether stitches are necessary:

- *Is the wound deep enough for subcutaneous (yellowish, fatty) tissue to be visible?* If yes, it is technically deep enough to require stitching.

- *Can the wound be pulled closed easily?* If not, stitches will be required to keep the wound closed for long enough to allow it to heal properly.

- *Where is the wound?* Wounds at locations of the body that move or stretch a lot will need stitches to stabilise and immobilise them long enough for self-repair.

SAVING A SEVERED BODY PART FOR REATTACHMENT

See the entries in the injuries section for specifics on digits, limbs, etc. (see pages 161, 166 and 168). Once bleeding is controlled at the site of the injury (via a dressing, pressure points, etc.) there may be an opportunity to save the severed body part for reattachment/replantation.

1. Gather up the amputated body part(s).

2. Place it/them inside a clean plastic bag that can be tied off to become water tight, or wrap small parts in cling film.

3. Place the bagged/wrapped body part(s) inside another bag filled with ice or packs of frozen vegetables.

4. Never put a severed limb directly onto ice as this can damage the tissues and complicate potential replantation.

INDEX OF PLANTS

(INCLUDING FUNCTIONAL FOOD AND KITCHEN HERBS/SPICES)

INDEX OF INJURIES

INDEX OF RECIPES